STOP

Trying to Lose Weight

You're Making Yourself

FATTER

STOP

Trying to Lose Weight

You're Making Yourself

FATTER

THE WAY TO A BETTER BODY IS NOT WHAT YOU THINK

Brian Murray

Stop Trying To Lose Weight You're Making Yourself Fatter
by Brian Murray

Library of Congress Cataloging in Publication data
Murray, Brian
Stop Trying To Lose Weight You're Making Yourself Fatter/Brian Murray.

ISBN 13: 978-0-9830075-2-4

Printed in the United States of America

This book is dedicated to my parents,
Paul and Janet Murray.

Acknowledgments

This book would not have been possible without the many dedicated clients who put forth a tremendous amount of effort over the past 12 years. I thank all of you.

A special thanks goes to Jeff Weinstock for urging me to restart my fat loss program and his wife Laura, who agreed to be the first participant. Laura impressed everyone with her commitment, dedication, and transformation. Laura's success encouraged many more people to participate and ultimately lead to the idea for this book. Thank you both for being the spark.

Thank you Melissa, Kylie, Shea, and Wynn. Your love and support inspire me to stay in the fight.

Most of all, I would like to thank my editor, Brenda Murray, for encouraging me to take on this project. Her insight and skill were invaluable and her constant guidance kept me focused on the most important steps of the process. Thank you for understanding when I didn't want to yield my position and for your commitment to getting this book published. This journey would not have been as much fun without you.

Contents

Introduction

How many times have you looked admiringly at someone in great shape and thought to yourself, "Wow, she has nice *weight*?" I bet never. You don't notice someone's weight. You notice bright eyes, healthy skin, muscle tone, pleasing shape, and the absence of excess fat. In other words, you notice characteristics that are attractive.

Your weight is not all that important to you. How do I know? Because no woman would care if she weighed 300 pounds if she were a firm and shapely size two. No man would care if he weighed 300 pounds if he had a 29-inch waist and chiseled abdominal muscles. So what are you really saying when you say, "I want to lose weight?" I bet that you are really saying, "I want to look attractive. I want to feel good about myself. I want to feel healthy, strong and confident; and I don't want to be fat."

The problem is, simply losing body weight will not get you there.

The title of this book is deliberately deceptive. Initially you may have thought, "What do you mean stop trying to lose weight? Have you seen me?" Yes, I have seen you, and if you have too much fat on your body of course I want you to lose weight, but I want you to lose the right kind of weight. Yes, there is a distinction. Not all weight loss is created equal. It can be good or bad, and the path that leads to not only the look you really want, but also the life you want, just may be the one less traveled. Getting on that path requires that you think differently.

Get Ready to Deprogram

"I feel like I'm cheating." This is what Natalie said to me when I checked her body composition after six weeks on my fat loss program. She lost 11 pounds of body fat, four inches off her waist, three inches off her hips, and three inches off her thighs without losing any lean body mass. She was eating better, sleeping more, resting more, and exercising less. Like you she had struggled in the past to lose weight. Now she couldn't believe she was losing fat, feeling great, and not *suffering* at the same time. I told her, "You aren't cheating. This is what it should feel like when you do it correctly. It should feel almost effortless."

Wouldn't you like to get more out of less? You wouldn't be alive if you didn't. So ask yourself this question: "Is it possible that nearly everything I think I know about losing weight and making my body more attractive is wrong?" Well of course it is; that's why I wrote this book.

For the past 12 years I have operated my own exercise

science laboratory. I have supervised thousands of exercise sessions and collected a wealth of clinical data on how the average person responds to a common sense approach to diet and exercise. I have helped hundreds of clients transform their bodies. As a result of this experience, one thing I can say with complete certainty is that pop-culture weight loss wisdom is wrong.

Since the very beginning my approach to helping people change their bodies has been consistently the same. Every person I put through my fat loss program is initially told, "You are going to do the exact opposite of everything you have been told about losing weight and getting in shape, and you will have better results for it." They eat more, but it's better quality food, exercise less, rest more, and never do one of the most devilish acts ever devised by man—cardio. Sounds impossible, right? Well, it's not, and this approach will beat any other approach hands down every time.

The Body Follows the Mind

The "experts" have certainly filled you with a wealth of misinformation. They have catered to your desire for the fantasy – you can have your cake and eat it too. Unfortunately, you have gobbled it all down and gotten nowhere.

I know you already know this, but I'm going to say it anyway. There is no such thing as a shortcut, so stop looking. They just don't exist. You have been told what you want to hear, not what you need to hear. This has confused you and compromised the results you could, or should have. This book will change that for you, if you choose to read this book with an open mind.

This book is not a presentation of my personal philosophy or trademarked system. What you are about to learn is reality; it is an exploration of the way the body really works, whether you like it or not. What you will read is based on a common sense understanding that you cannot break the laws of nature; you can only surrender to them in order to produce the changes you want. Basically, I'm just pointing out the truth to you, and I make no apologies for doing it. Even though the truth is often painful, the truth is the only thing that will set you free from poor results, frustration, and confusion.

This book is designed to change the way you think, not your behavior. There's a big difference. If you're like most you probably blame your physique problems on your family tree, your age, your thyroid or your exercise program, when all you need to do is point the blame where it should be – your head. You fight yourself in your mind. I want to help you stop that, but it requires thinking in a manner opposite of everything you believe to be true.

I give you permission to indulge your inner contrarian—the one who knows there's got to be a better way than the ones that exercise pundits preach. If you can open yourself to a new way of thinking and break old patterns, you'll find that you've been right all along! After reading this book you will be able to drive by the gym without guilt that you aren't there. You will snicker at the tips and tricks for "losing the last five pounds" on the covers of magazines. You will think twice before considering permanently mutilating your body with life-threatening surgery. You will be happier and have more time for yourself and the things you really want to do. Most importantly, you will stop letting your bathroom scale determine your mood for the day.

Who Is This Book For?

This book is for everyone with a body. It is for you, the person who erroneously thinks your body weight is important, the person who wishes there was a better way, or the person who is sick and tired of getting nowhere and would like to break the chains of confusion and frustration. If you've tried everything, worked really hard, felt like you've killed yourself to be thin, read every magazine article on weight loss, and tried every diet with no luck, this book will help light a new and more rewarding path to follow.

"But what if I have 100 pounds to lose?" you ask.

My answer: it doesn't matter if you have 1, 10, or 100 pounds to lose. The approach I am advocating for will work. This book is for the person who wants to change a little or a lot. Don't look at the before and after pictures in this book and say "she was in shape already!" You've just set yourself up for failure. You've just counted yourself out when you shouldn't have. You're human and the laws of nature that I'll explain to you apply to every human, regardless of the amount of change that's required.

You are going to learn something new that will help you get where you want to be, but don't expect a bunch of photos showing step by step exercise instructions and a list of menus and recipes. Although these would give you a concrete plan to follow, you don't need them. I'm going to give you something much more valuable: a new way of thinking, new thought patterns, and a new framework for living your life. Read on. Your life is about to change forever.

CHAPTER ONE

Bad Weight Loss

*So you lost 20 pounds. Big deal. You
just made yourself fatter.*

You did it the old-fashioned way. You ate less and exercised more, or maybe not at all. The part about eating less is good. Obviously you were eating too much and without a calorie cutback your fat cells wouldn't even think about shrinking. But the exercise part is a big problem. Nevertheless, your goal was weight loss, and you succeeded, but at the expense of your health, appearance, and sanity, now and into the future.

You are now 20 pounds *lighter*, but what have you really lost? Are you 20 pounds *leaner*? Your bathroom scale is clueless, you are too, and that's good for business. The weight loss industry depends on you not understanding that two things help your weight loss and undermine your health, appearance, and ability to keep the weight off long-term—dehydration and loss of lean body mass. That's right. It's all a very lucrative illusion and the less you know the better.

Brian Murray

The fact is there is little evidence that commercial weight loss systems are effective, and the companies that sell those systems are not interested in conducting studies to prove they are. In a *New York Times* article titled "Diet and Lose Weight? Scientists Say 'Prove It!,'" Richard Cleland, assistant director for advertising practices at the Federal Trade Commission says, "In general, the industry has always been opposed to making outcomes disclosures. They have always given various rationales from 'It's too expensive,' to even arguing that part of this is selling the dream, and if you know what the truth is, it's harder to sell the dream." Busted! It's much easier to separate you from your money when you don't know the truth. But honestly, the industry doesn't even know what the truth is. I do and now you will too.

When the paid spokesperson for the diet plan proclaims "I lost 40 pounds in 8 weeks!" you should know that those 40 pounds are comprised of mostly water and lean body mass—two of your most important assets. To understand this you need to know what makes up your weight.

The human body is really nothing more than an organized bag of seawater. Three basic categories comprise your total weight: fluid, lean tissues (primarily muscle), and fat. Water makes up almost 70 percent of your total mass. Water and lean tissue are much denser than fat and, volume for volume, weigh much more than fat. Lean tissue also has higher water content than fat. Can you now see why losing water and lean body mass lead to a much bigger chunk of weight loss? They are heavier.

Most of your water volume is included in your lean body mass. When you lose a lot of weight as fluid, it is pulled from within your muscle cells and from blood plasma. This is not good because you reduce the energy producing capability of your cells, and therefore the proper functioning of your body.

The average American experiences symptoms of dehydration after losing just one percent of body weight as water (about two percent of normal water volume). If you weigh 200 pounds this equates to just two pounds, but you probably won't even notice how damaging this can be. If you are like most, you have been dehydrated for years and have lived with dry skin, heart palpitations, headaches, constipation, joint pain, muscle spasms, fatigue, and irritability for so long that the symptoms of the condition seem normal.

Now let's go back to the 20 pounds you lost. What you really lost was a combination of 18 pounds of water and lean body mass—muscle, bone, organ tissue, and nerve tissue, whatever. If it was good stuff you lost it. This is *bad weight loss*.

Basically, you have just thrown the baby out with the bath water. To lose anything other than fat is a serious insult to your vitality and appearance. Sure, you will get attention for the change in your size, but is it really worth compromising your health to make it happen? Apparently, the answer is yes. In a survey conducted by Harvard Medical School internist Dr. Christina Wee, 19 percent of overweight people and 33 percent of obese people would risk death for even a modest 10-pound weight loss. These same people were also willing to give up some of their remaining years of life if they could live those years weighing slightly less.

Be careful what you wish for. Analysis of time to death in two population-based studies, the Tecumseh Community Health Study (1,890 subjects) and the Framingham Heart Study (2,731 subjects), found that regardless of the statistical approach used, weight loss was associated with *increased* mortality rate while fat loss was associated with *decreased* mortality rate. It looks like your desire to lose weight may be a death wish.

Now back to you and your weight loss. You have just made it next to impossible to keep the weight off and avoid gaining even more fat in the future. Why? Your muscle mass and all other lean tissues account for a large portion of your resting metabolic rate. You lost some of those tissues and now your resting metabolic rate is going to decline at a much faster rate than it naturally should. This is where exercise plays a very important role, but not just any form of activity; it must be the right type of exercise to prevent this from happening.

Ironically, the same two things that help your weight

loss—dehydration and loss of lean body mass—also *hurt* your fat loss; the stuff you really want to get rid of. You may think that weight loss equals fat loss, but it doesn't. A recent study conducted by Louisiana State University researcher and chair in Health Wisdom, Dr. Timothy Church, found that out of three groups of overweight women who exercised for various weekly durations for six months, the group that exercised the most each week lost an average of only 3.3 pounds of body weight, of which only *two-tenths* was from body fat. Does a loss of two-tenths of a pound of body fat after six months of hours of exercise each week sound rewarding to you? I didn't think so.

Now let's return again to the 20 pounds you lost. Only two pounds were from body fat. Why so little? You ate less and exercised like a maniac. With all that exercise, shouldn't you have lost more fat? No. Here's why: your brain relied on ancient survival programming and thought, "I'm being chased by a tiger and there isn't enough food to replenish all the energy I'm expending." Basically, your body felt threatened, so it kept fat around just in case you lived and the food supply wasn't plentiful. Besides, it's easier for your body to keep fat around. It has a whopping metabolic rate of two calories per pound, so it doesn't cost your body much to carry it.

On the other hand, muscle is active tissue with a much higher metabolic rate, at least three times that of fat. It is metabolically expensive to carry and your body is a master of economics. If you do not challenge your muscles, especially during the initial stage of a weight loss program, your body does not perceive a need to keep them, so your muscles become expendable and wither away as they are burned for fuel. Again, this can all be avoided with the right type of exercise, but if you think all that walking and jogging will help, think again. It doesn't challenge your muscles the way you need it to. It's passively making you fatter.

I know what you're thinking. "How can I lose 20 pounds, drop two sizes, and possibly be fatter?" Not only is it possible, it's what often happens when you focus on your body weight and fail to consider what has happened to your body composition—your fat mass and lean body mass.

Again, we visit the 20 pounds you lost, but view it in the context of how it affected your body composition.

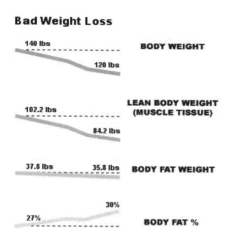

What we see is that the lean body mass component of your body represented a large portion of your weight loss while a small portion was represented by your fat mass component. This means that your fat mass now represents a larger *percent-*

Figure 1 The chart above shows how you can make yourself fatter even if you reduce your body weight.

age of your body weight than it did before you lost weight. So even though your jeans now fit a little looser, you have made yourself a fatter, softer, weaker, less healthy, and more injury-prone person. Sure you are lighter, but now you are just a smaller version of a fat person. But the worst is yet to come.

Sadly, you are now heading for a ride on the weight loss/fat gain roller coaster without a seatbelt. Sooner or later you are going to go off your diet, and when you do the weight is coming back with a vengeance. What comes back is a lot of FAT. The portion of your body composition represented by fat goes up and the lean body mass component doesn't change from its now further reduced level. Your body fat percentage climbs even higher! So the next time you muster enough willpower to "lose weight" your battle is going to be even tougher, and you will fail to improve your body… again.

This is the story of millions of people: a story of frustration, discouragement, and unhappiness. It doesn't have to be this way. There can be a happy ending; you can live happily ever after.

My good friend and Identity Therapy expert, Dr. Lynn Seiser says, "There are no problems, only solutions that don't work." You need a new solution. I've got one for you. But first you've got a lot to unlearn.

CHAPTER TWO

Master of Disguise

Are you overweight, or overfat and undermuscled?

In case you haven't noticed, blue jeans do not have weight limits. A 150-pound lady with 25 pounds of fat on her body can easily wear the size four that a 135-pound lady with 40 pounds of fat could not get past her thighs. Why? The 150-pound lady has a lot less fat and a lot more muscle. The point? Body weight doesn't matter. How much space you occupy does, and this is dependent upon the *quality* of your body composition.

Your body has three basic components: water, lean body mass (including muscle, organs, nerves and bones) and fat. These components can be divided into two broad categories: lean body mass and fat mass. The shape of your body at any time in your life is determined by three things: your bones, muscles, and degree of fatness.

Your skeleton is simply a hanger on which everything else rests. You cannot change the shape of your skeleton. Therefore, the state of your muscles—flabby or firm—and the size of your fat cells determine your contours. The good news is that you can alter the *quantity* of these tissues through diet and exercise.

If muscle and fat determine your basic contours, why are you watching your weight? Your weight doesn't tell you anything about how much muscle or fat you have. Weight loss doesn't mean fat loss. You can lose weight and still gain fat and lose muscle. You can gain weight and still lose fat while gaining muscle. Not all weight gain is bad weight gain. Not all weight loss is good weight loss.

Watching your weight is deceptive. This is where your struggle begins. So what should you be watching? You need to watch what is happening to the muscle and fat content of your body. Failure to track your muscle-to-fat ratio will mean your efforts to truly improve your appearance will most likely fail.

Your muscle-to-fat ratio is a comparison of the number of pounds of muscle on your body to the number of pounds of fat. When it comes to improving your health, appearance, and self-esteem this should be your primary concern, not your weight. Maximum muscle and a healthy amount of fat determine a beautiful body, not a body weight of 110 pounds.

Dr. Ellington Darden, former director of research for Nautilus Sports/Medical Industries and highly acclaimed fitness expert has authored several books on the subject of fat loss. His data reveals shocking changes to the muscle to fat ratio that occur in the average female as she ages.

At age 14 she is at her muscular peak. She weighs approximately 120 pounds and has 48 pounds of muscle and

20 pounds of fat. Her muscle/fat ratio is 48:20, or 2.4 to 1. This means that she has 2.4 pounds of muscle for every pound of fat. She is lean, firm, and shapely. But with each year that passes she loses a half-pound of muscle and gains 1.5 pounds of fat.

Fast forward to age 50. She has now gained approximately 36 pounds. Her muscle decreased by 18 pounds and her fat increased by 54 pounds. Her muscle/fat ratio is now 30:74, or 1 to 2.4, which means that for every pound of muscle she now has 2.4 pounds of fat. This is a complete reversal, and her body fat percentage increased by nearly 300 percent!

If this woman thinks she is only 36 pounds overweight she better think again. She is really 54 pounds overfat and 18 pounds undermuscled. You are in the same boat, yet you continue to focus on how much you weigh. The scale is duping you!

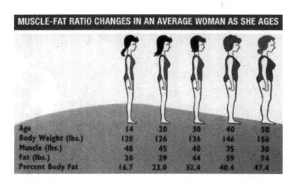

MUSCLE-FAT RATIO CHANGES IN AN AVERAGE WOMAN AS SHE AGES

Age	14	20	30	40	50
Body Weight (lbs.)	120	126	136	146	156
Muscle (lbs.)	48	45	40	35	30
Fat (lbs.)	20	29	44	59	74
Percent Body Fat	16.7	23.0	32.4	40.4	47.4

Figure 2 As we age, loss of muscle mass is a major factor in fat gain. Illustration from *Body Defining* by Ellington Darden. Published by McGraw Hill, 1996. Reproduced with permission of the McGraw Hill Companies.

Your weight gain is a symptom of a much larger problem. You must ask yourself, "What is it that I am gaining that is making my weight go up?" As you can see from the preceding example, you are gaining massive amounts of fat. Why? Loss of muscle mass is a major factor.

In their 1991 bestseller *Biomarkers*, Dr. William Evans and Dr. Irwin Rosenberg present their findings from many studies conducted at the USDA Nutrition Research Center on Aging at Tufts University. The authors identify ten biomarkers, or key physiological factors associated with prolonged youth and vitality. Care to guess what the number one biomarker of aging is? Muscle mass.

The research clearly demonstrates that the age related loss of muscle mass is the lead domino in a long lineup of biomarkers. As muscle mass topples a cascade of negative events occur within the body, the most noticeable is the accumulation of excess fat.

Many long-term studies show that as we move from our physical peak in young adulthood to middle age we lose almost seven pounds of lean body mass every decade, and that this rate of loss accelerates after the age of 45. Why? That brings us to the number two biomarker of aging—strength.

We simply don't challenge our muscles anymore, and this is bad for our muscle-to-fat ratio. But the process of losing muscle and gaining fat is sneaky. Muscle loss proceeds at such a slow rate that you don't notice what is happening until one day you realize you look and feel 20 years older than you really are. The good news is that you can reverse this process. You can reclaim the muscles of your youth, or if you are still young, prevent this from ever occurring. However, you are going to have to get stronger.

One thing is certain: you don't have too much weight, you have too much fat, too little muscle, and your body weight disguises the severity of your deteriorating figure.

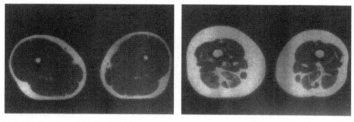

Figure 3 PROPORTION OF LEAN BODY MASS VERSUS FAT IN YOUNG AND OLDER WOMEN. These two magnetic resonance images make a dramatic point about the loss of lean body mass and the accumulation of fat as we age. Both show a cross-sectional view of a woman's thigh. The top photo is the thigh of a 20 year old athlete. The bottom is the thigh of a sedentary 64 year old woman. The young woman has a body mass index (BMI) of 22.6; the older woman, a BMI of 30.7. Reprinted with the permission of Fireside an imprint of Simon & Schuster, Inc., from *BIOMARKERS: The 10 Keys to Prolonging Vitality* by Williams Evans, Ph.D and Irwin H. Rosenberg, M.D. Copyright © 1991 by Dr. Irwin H. Rosenberg, Dr. William J. Evans, and Jacqueline Thompson. All rights reserved.

Your scale is enabling you to live in denial. I realized this one day when I collected body composition measurements from a new client. She had been a long time member of *Weight Watchers*® and had recently gotten serious about losing weight... again. The only thing she had ever measured was her body weight so she had no idea what might be happening under her skin, yet she knew the numbers were not going to be good. They weren't.

I asked if her reading surprised her. She wasn't. She said, "You already know the information is going to be bad. You think what you don't know won't hurt you. It's avoidance of guilt." Perhaps that is why we are so fixated on our weight – it doesn't tell us what we need to know and allows us to avoid discomfort.

Well, the cold hard truth is that you will never improve yourself by staying in your comfort zone. You need to know what is happening inside your body no matter how unpleasant the information may be. Acknowledging the problem is the first step toward correcting it.

Telling yourself that you need to lose weight is not the same as telling yourself that you need to lose fat and gain muscle.

If you believe you only need to lose weight, then you don't have to think about losing fat and gaining muscle. See how easy that is? This is why weight watching is your primary focus; it's easy, the feedback is immediate, and it requires little thought and planning. Losing fat and gaining muscle requires more thought, patience, and discipline on the front end, but the end results are more rewarding and longer lasting.

Your body weight is a meaningless number. Let it go. You need more information.

CHAPTER THREE

Weight is for Suckers

What does your bathroom scale tell you?
Absolutely nothing of any value.

When someone tells me they lost 10 pounds I like to ask "Ten pounds of what?" Of course they can't answer the question—they don't know what they *really* lost, and to their detriment, often don't care. I realized this one day when I stopped a woman who was briskly walking around my office building. I wanted to give her a promotional postcard for my six-week fat loss program. As I handed her the postcard I asked if she was out for a "fitness walk" and she said yes, and told me that she had lost 18 pounds. I replied, "Eighteen pounds of what?" to which she replied, "I don't know but it's gone."

You should know what you are losing.

Weight loss is meaningless unless the *quality* of the weight can be stated. Did you lose water? Fat? Muscle? Your mind? If you don't know what you are losing or gaining how do you know if what you are doing or not doing is working for you or against you?

You need more information.

For the past four years I have collected body composition data on clients using a Tanita® Body Composition Monitor. It calculates body composition using Bioelectrical Impedance Analysis (BIA). A safe, low-level electrical signal is passed through the body. Electricity passes easily through fluids in the muscle and other body tissues but meets resistance as it passes through body fat, which contains little fluid. When used under consistent conditions this device gives you the information you need to evaluate what is actually happening to your body as a result of exercise or dietary modifications. You should be primarily interested in how your measurements trend over time. The following scenarios indicate that you are getting leaner:

Scenario 1: Body fat percentage goes down while muscle mass goes up

Scenario 2: Body fat percentage goes down while muscle mass remains the same.

Scenario 3: Muscle mass goes up, body fat does not change.

In keeping with weight being the great master of disguise, in scenarios 1 and 3, your body weight could be going up. Hence, not all weight gain is bad.

Sadly, you watch your body weight, which is meaningless, and for you to be happy the number can only go one way—down. But wouldn't it be nice if it were a good thing

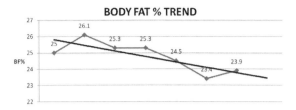

Figure 5 In the chart above, the last measurement is higher than the previous measurement yet the overall trend was still downward. Remember, the overall trend is what is important, not the individual measurements. Your body weight cannot give you this information.

if the number didn't change or even went up? Instead of being happy with only one outcome, you could now be happy with several different outcomes. The chart above shows how measurements can go up, down, or stay the same over time. This is normal and to be expected. Regardless of what happens, and what the actual numbers are, your goal is to see a downward trend in body fat percentage.

To illustrate how meaningless your body weight is, and the true story behind it, I will share with you Pat's quarterly body composition data over the past three years. I'm going to throw some numbers at you, but what I really want you to pay attention to is how the change in Pat's body composition accounted for his change in body weight. By the way, Pat's age during these measurements was 50, 51, and 52. All of these measurements were taken at 12:20 p.m. on Wednesday afternoons:

Measurement 1

Between measurements for the first and second quarter of 2006, Pat's body weight does not change. Looking beyond weight at what is really important—muscle and fat—we see that his lean body mass increases 3.5 pounds while his body fat drops by 3.5 pounds. Body weight did not change. Body composition changed for the better. Pat is now leaner.

Measurement 2

Between the second and third quarter of 2006, Pat loses six pounds of body weight, but the change in his body composition is even more dramatic. His lean body mass increases by six pounds while his body fat decreases by 12 pounds! His lean body mass as a percentage of his body weight has risen from 63 percent to 68 percent. Pat is now even leaner.

Measurement 3

Between the fourth quarter of 2006 and the second quarter of 2007 Pat's body weight does not change much at all; just a little over one pound. For many this would be a huge victory to make it through the holiday season without gaining 10 pounds, however, it's not as good as it seems. Pat gained 3.7 pounds of fat while losing 2.4 pounds of lean body mass. His lean body mass now represents only 65 percent of his body weight. Pat is now a little fatter.

Measurement 4

Between the second and third quarter of 2007 Pat's

body weight goes down by 2.6 pounds. However, his lean body mass goes up by 3.3 pounds while his body fat goes down by six pounds! Again, there is a small change in body weight but a big change in body composition. His lean body mass now represents 67 percent of his body weight. Pat is now leaner.

Measurement 5

Between the third and fourth quarter of 2007 Pat's body weight does not change at all. Knowing that body weight is the great deceiver, we look further and find that he has gained 4.1 pounds of fat and lost 4.1 pounds of lean body mass. Lean body mass as a percentage of body weight decreases slightly.

Measurement 6

Pat packs on the pounds this holiday season. Between the fourth quarter of 2007 and the first quarter of 2008 Pat gains seven pounds of body weight. But what did he really gain? It turns out that he only gained a measly half-pound of body fat. The rest was lean body mass. So was the weight gain bad? No.

A New Perspective

During the past three years Pat's body weight has fluctuated up and down. Today it is nearly identical to what it was three years ago. To the weight-watcher this would probably be disappointing, but for Pat it's not. He is three years older, however, he now carries eight pounds LESS body fat and eight pounds MORE lean body mass. Wouldn't you love to see your body composition improve as you get older?

As you can clearly see, your body weight doesn't tell you what is really going on. Yet, even after teaching this to people year after year they still can't let go of this simple and quick number. I still hear the groans of anxiety when a new quarter rolls around and it's time to check body composition. Why? Everyone is worried about his or her weight. The first number that pops up on the monitor is their body weight. If it doesn't go down, they react with a sigh of disappointment. Yet when I tell them, for example, that they had a three-pound fat loss and a three-pound lean body mass gain, they reply, "Oh that makes me feel better."

Why the need to feel bad in the first place? Get a body composition monitor and look deeper into what is really happening to your body. More information about your body composition will not only free you from disappointment, but give you the feedback you need to make the adjustments necessary to keep your body composition moving in the right direction.

Still want to lose weight? No you don't. You want to lose fat and gain muscle. You want good weight loss.

CHAPTER FOUR

Good Weight Loss

Imagine this. You lose 10 pounds of body weight, but you look and feel like you lost 20. How?

It all started with a new mindset. You didn't care about your body weight and your first priority was watching your muscle and fat changes. You made the usual dietary changes—portion control and healthier food choices—and combined that with the right type of exercise, which you will soon learn is the secret ingredient in your recipe for success.

Your goal was to lose fat, and only fat. While you were reducing your dietary calories you performed exercise that forced your body to keep all the good stuff—muscle, bone, organ, nerve tissues, and vital fluids—while you lost only fat. This *targeted fat loss* broadcasts attractiveness and is essential for maintaining the striking results you earned well into the future. However, the only way to guarantee fat loss was by making your muscles work against a lot of resistance.

With the right type of exercise you stimulated your muscles to become younger and more energetic, using excess fat as a source of energy for growth and strength improvement. This also forced valuable, youth-preserving fluids to stay in your muscles and blood plasma to help with the transport of nutrients and hormones, removal of waste, and the survival of every cell in your body.

Since you abandoned weight watching, you tracked your muscle and fat changes on your body composition monitor and noticed that you gained two pounds of muscle. But wait; didn't you also lose 10 pounds of body weight? How do you gain and lose at the same time? What happened?

The addition of those two extra pounds of highly active calorie-burning muscle tissue helped vaporize 12 pounds of body fat! Yes, you did it the right way and the pounds of fat you lost were greater than the pounds of body weight you lost because you gained muscle and guaranteed that everything you lost was fat. This is good weight loss.

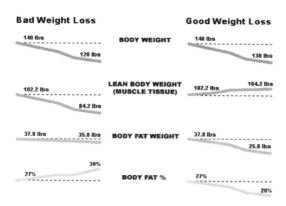

Figure 5 Both people above start with the same body weight and fat percentage. However, the person with good weight loss drops 10 pounds of body weight and ends with a body fat percentage 10 points lower than the person who lost 20 pounds of body weight.

See, gaining weight isn't all that bad after all. When you think differently and focus on what you need to gain instead of what you struggle to lose, the most overlooked and underappreciated secret weapon for fighting fat becomes apparent—gain muscle to lose fat. This is how you keep fat off PERMANENTLY!

The beautiful thing about what you accomplished is that all of your weight loss was fat loss, something that doesn't occur when you employ conventional weight loss methods. Also, you did not sacrifice any part of your body with joint crippling cardio activities, or compromise your health with further dehydration or muscle loss. Your new muscle to fat ratio changed your appearance dramatically, yet you didn't lose a lot of weight.

Now, I understand that you have been in a long-term serious relationship and it may take you a while to break up with your body weight. I know I won't get any endorsements from *Weight Watchers*® or *Jenny Craig*®, and I hate to disappoint you, but you will not be the one pictured in the testimonial claiming you lost the equivalent of a fourth-grader in eight weeks. With this new approach you didn't need to lose a lot of weight. Here's why.

You kept your muscles and vital fluids—the heavier substances in your body. Muscle is firm, smooth, shapely, and wraps tightly to your skeleton. You lost fat. Fat is formless, lumpy and bumpy, and it hangs off your body. Did you catch that? It hangs. That isn't a good look for fat, especially when you have more than you should. And if you were to look at three pounds of fat next to three pounds of muscle the fat takes up TWICE the space. Did you get that? TWICE the space. Now tell me, which would you rather wear?

Think of it this way. If your body weight does not change and you gain three pounds of muscle, you are leaner because your body fat represents a smaller percentage of your body weight. The additional muscle also smoothes out dimpled skin and gives you more pleasing curves. On the other hand, if you lose three pounds of fat your silhouette becomes smaller, your muscle represents a higher percentage of your body weight, and you are leaner. But if you lose fat AND gain muscle *at the same time* the change in your muscle to fat ratio and effect on your appearance is striking.

This is called *synergy*.

The simultaneous occurrences of reducing calorie intake, hydrating your system, and the right type of exercise together create a greater total effect than each one would separately. In other words, one plus one plus one equals six!

Doesn't this sound like a much more rewarding approach to getting the look you want and being able to maintain it forever? Of course. Take this approach from now on. Be lean, strong, happy and confident, forever.

Trust me, if every person with too much fat on their body took this approach, the obesity epidemic would reverse itself several fold within six months.

It's time for a revolution. Let's scrap the old way of doing things and start over. Are you with me? If so, you are going to have to change the way you think about exercise.

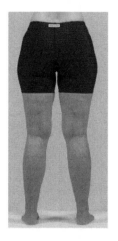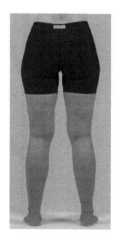

Figure 6 The person in the before and after photos above lost 10.5 pounds of fat in six weeks. Look at the effect: a noticeable reduction of the hips and thighs, a smoothing effect, and a firmer appearance. This is good weight loss.

CHAPTER FIVE

Walking Is Not Exercise

You could walk all the way from Manhattan to Malibu and not improve your muscle to fat ratio. In fact, it would become worse.

Everywhere you look people are walking. We walk from our cars into stores. We walk while we work, while we shop, and even while we eat. The fact is, we do a lot of walking, and we have walked a lot since the day we took our first steps. Have we become more muscular and less fat with age? No. So why is walking touted as the best form of exercise?

The truth is you know walking is not the best form of exercise. Unfortunately, you may not trust your instincts because of social pressure. I will help you completely understand why walking is not exercise.

Although he does not come to mind when you consider pioneers of exercise, Leonardo Da Vinci's drawings of human anatomy demonstrated the relationship between the bones as levers and the muscles as the engines that produce human movement. When you understand how the bony levers and muscles work together you will know why walking is not productive exercise.

While standing, bend your knees slightly, hold that position, and note the difficulty. How long could you hold this position? A very long time. Now stand with your back against a wall and move your feet approximately 18-24 inches away from the wall. Slowly bend your knees and slide your body down the wall until your thighs are parallel to the floor. Hold this position and note the difficulty. How long do you think you could hold this position? If you can tolerate intense muscle burn, maybe two minutes.

Now you understand leverage, and why walking will never improve your body composition—it's too easy. It doesn't deeply fatigue your muscles.

Results vs. Effects

If you want a great body, fat loss and muscle gain should be your goal. The right type of exercise can help the process along efficiently. The wrong type of exercise will help you get fatter and weaker, so if you are going to spend your valuable time exercising it is in your best interest to think about what you really want to get in return for your effort.

Do you want results or effects?

The term *result* means a long-term change in muscular strength, firmness, and shape, bone strength, leanness, and an overall improvement of physical capability. The term *effect* means the immediate change in the body's homeostasis because of movement, such as increased heart rate, labored breathing, sweating, and light muscle fatigue.

Effects and results are both consequences, but an effect is an immediate consequence, while a result is a consequence that occurs after several days or weeks. In other words, results require patience.

Effects are fleeting. When you stop exercising the effects usually subside within several minutes. Results are more long lasting. Once you gain them it takes a much longer time to lose them. This makes sense. If your body is going to expend energy to coordinate the building of new tissues over the course of several weeks, it isn't going to turn around and tear it all down overnight. For example, in a study from the University of Maryland, both men and women were subjected to strength training of the frontal thigh muscles for nine weeks followed by no strength training of the same muscles for 31 weeks. The researchers assessed muscle quality, which was defined as the maximum amount of force the muscles could produce per unit of muscle mass. The muscle quality assessment took place at baseline, after nine weeks of strength training, and after 31 weeks of detraining.

All subjects exhibited significantly increased strength and muscle volume after the nine-week training period. So what would you expect to see after 31 weeks of no strength training for the thigh muscles? Would their results have vanished completely? No. Even after 31 weeks of no strengthening exercise the muscle quality of the thighs was still significantly elevated above baseline measurements.

Please sear the following deeply into your brain. Just because you are experiencing exercise effects doesn't mean you are going to get results from your exercise. Unfortunately, this is most likely why you continue to walk and jog with little to show for it—you are in love with the effects and most likely believe that the effects translate into results. Sweating equals fat loss, right? A little muscle fatigue equals more shapely muscles, right? Wrong.

Repetitive dumbbell pumping for the arms and never ending, knee-pounding activities like walking, jogging, and other activities categorized as cardio or aerobic workouts are high on effects but low on results. In his book *Hold It! You're Exercising Wrong*, author Edward Jackowski states, "I interviewed over a thousand women…and asked them 'How many women, including yourself, do you know who have ever vastly improved their body by taking aerobics classes?' All of them said zero, not one!"

So what do you want? A few temporary physiological changes that will be gone in a few minutes so you can start all over again tomorrow, or do you want your body to experience a permanent change that will make you look and feel twenty years younger all the time?

The effects may feel good, but it's the results that ultimately make you look better.

The First Step toward Results

One of the first things I tell clients during consultations is that the workout I am about to put them through produces absolutely no benefit to their body. It can't. The workout is the means to the end, not the end itself. In other words, your workout can stimulate your body to change. Only your body can *produce* those changes.

The simplest analogy is getting a tan. In order to develop a darker skin tone you must expose your skin to ultraviolet radiation. If the exposure is intense enough to threaten your body, it will change skin pigment to protect itself against another exposure. This change usually happens over the course of a few days. The sun doesn't produce the tan, your body does. Your skin would have become darker even if you had stayed indoors for three days after you were out in the sun.

The same thing works with exercise. If you want your body to upgrade its capability—stronger bones, stronger muscles, and improved cardiovascular efficiency—you must threaten it; make it feel inadequate. If your exercise is intense enough to threaten your body, and you give your body some time to rest, it will make itself even more capable over the course of a few days.

The problem is that your body does not like to change, so you have to give it a good reason to change. That is why it takes a high degree of muscular effort to make this happen. In other words, your exercise must be intense. It must produce a deep level of fatigue in a short period of time. My clients understand this concept; it is a fatigue that makes their legs so shaky they feel the need to rest a few extra minutes before attempting to drive away.

Exercise is simply a tool to encourage your body to change for the better. To get the changes you want you must exert muscular effort above and beyond what your body is accustomed to every time you exercise, otherwise your body will keep marching in the direction of deterioration.

Your muscles are the window to your body. Your entire physiological apparatus exists to support what your muscles do—produce movement. Exercise that taxes your muscles deeply will lead to improvement of all the systems in your body. Therefore, your exercise should lead to improved muscle strength, and this is best accomplished by putting your muscles in a mechanically disadvantageous position.

Humans graduate from crawling to walking because walking is the most efficient form of human movement. In other words, walking places our muscles in a mechanically advantageous position so fatigue does not occur. Can you imagine how tiring it would be to have to crawl everywhere you went?

The question is, if your body will only upgrade its capability if you ask it to exert effort beyond what is normal, and walking is the easiest and least energy-consuming form of movement, how can walking help your muscle to fat ratio? It can't. It will not lead to stronger muscles. That means you will gain body fat as time goes by.

Don't get me wrong, I have nothing against walking,

but don't walk and expect a better body. It's great for effects, not for results that will make a *real* difference in your life. Walk for enjoyment and transportation, not for exercise. It's too easy.

CHAPTER SIX

Life in a Fool's Paradise

You walk. You jog. You do your cardio. You do this a lot because it "burns calories." Really? If you go to the American College of Sports Medicine meeting this year and ask 100 exercise physiologists their opinion, every one of them will tell you there is nothing more wildly exaggerated than people's estimates of the number of calories they burn during exercise.

When it comes to burning calories the first thing you need to understand is that you are locked in a battle with Mother Nature. You are fighting millions of years of evolutionary biology. Our physiological systems developed for one purpose—survival. You can't win. You won't win.

Increased caloric expenditure from exercise is so far down the list of factors contributing to fat loss that it barely makes the list, yet this is probably your number one reason for enduring such mindless activity. The fact is you will burn a few calories, but hardly enough to make it worth your time. Like every other living thing on this planet your body is hardwired to *conserve* energy, not expend energy. No human would have survived this long if that wasn't the case.

So you continue your walk or jog comforted by the thought of the 300 calories you will have burned after your hour of cardio is complete. Dream on.

Let's say you are the average size female. According to the Centers for Disease Control and Prevention that would make you 5'4" tall with a body weight of 163 pounds. Let's make you 40 years old. According to the *Discovery Health* website your basal metabolic rate would be 1,469 calories per day, or 61 calories per hour. This is the minimum number of calories you would expend each day if you did nothing. In other words, these are calories you are going to expend no matter what you do. So are you really going to expend 300 calories in one hour? No. You must subtract the calories you are going to burn anyway. This means the best you can hope for is 239 calories above your resting metabolism, if you're lucky.

At this point you may be thinking, "Well, 239 calories still isn't bad". Are you sure? It will require one hour of your time to expend those calories, and that is assuming you are moving at a very vigorous pace, something you probably don't do. So most likely you will not even burn 239 calories. But there is something else you may not account for. Kinesiologists call it *economy of motion*.

In a 2007 *New York Times* article titled "Putting Very Little Weight in Calorie Counting Methods," author Gina Kolata cites the work of Dr. Claude Bouchard, an obesity and exercise researcher who directs the Pennington Biomedical Research Center in Baton Rouge, Louisiana. He had subjects ride stationary bicycles six days a week for 12 weeks. At the end of the study they were burning 10 percent fewer calories at the same given level of effort. "The reason is that people perform an exercise more efficiently as they become more accustomed to it," said Dr. Bouchard.

I've seen you. You are accustomed all right. You "punch the cardio clock" a few days a week doing your same jog for the same distance at the same pace—slow. The calories you burn tomorrow are not going to be the same as the calories you burn today. If you are going to burn more calories you will have to add another 20 minutes each time out. Is that how you really want to spend your time? I'm going to guess not. But it gets worse. Care to guess what happens to your appetite?

Dr. Richard Cooper, chairman of the Department of Preventive Medicine and Epidemiology at Loyola University states, "People burn more calories when they exercise. Thing is, they compensate by eating more." So we must consider this question: could exercise be making it harder for you to slim down?

In the August 2009 issue of *Time*, author John Cloud addresses that question in his article titled "Why Exercise Won't Make You Thin." In the article he cites an interesting study by Louisiana State University Exercise Researcher and Chair in Health Wisdom Dr. Timothy Church. Dr. Church assigned 464 overweight and obese women who did not regularly exercise into four groups. Three of the groups participated in supervised exercise for 72 minutes, 136 minutes, and 194 minutes per week, respectively, for six months. The fourth group served as a non-exercising control. All groups were asked not to change their normal dietary habits. The results may surprise you.

On average, all groups lost a small amount of weight, but the groups that exercised, plodding along on a recumbent bike and treadmill several minutes a week for *six months* did not lose much more weight than the group that didn't do any exercise. So what happened here? Cloud writes, "Church calls it compensation, but you and I might know it as the lip-licking anticipation of perfectly salted, golden-brown french fries after a hard trip to the gym. Whether because exercise made them hungry or because they wanted to reward themselves (or both), most of the women who exercised ate more than they did before they started the experiment."

Now back to you. After your hour is finished and you "reward" yourself with a buttered bagel and latte, you will take in 600 calories or more in less than 15 minutes! Now if it were possible to burn off 600 calories in 15 minutes I would say bon appetite, but it's not possible. Now you have not only cancelled the extra calories you burned, but left yourself with a huge calorie surplus, and that was your one and only workout for the day! How, pray tell, are you going to "offset" all of your other meals for the day?

I hope it is now clear why exercising to burn off the excess calories you ingest is a losing proposition. If it hasn't occurred to you that you don't have to burn off what you don't put in your mouth, I hope this helps. Mark my words; it is the only way to win this game.

Relying on exercise to burn calories won't solve your issues. Knowing this, you'll have to focus on what *really* makes your jeans tighter—your eating habits.

CHAPTER SEVEN

You Eat Too Much

For someone with a diametrically opposing approach, I was always looking for ways to more effectively communicate my message. Going "behind enemy lines" and learning how obese people think only seemed logical. So several years ago I watched one of the post-weight loss interviews on the reality television show *The Biggest Loser*.

I wasn't disappointed.

What the interviewee said was so obvious. Millions of people must think this way. Why didn't I think of this before? It was so concise that I quickly grabbed a pen and wrote her statement word for word—"*I would rather exercise more than change the way I eat.*"

My first thought was, "Lady, it's never going to work. You will always be fat."

Let's be honest. We all know it. We wish it weren't true and I know you don't want to hear this, but the sooner you accept it the sooner you can start to successfully lose fat and keep it off permanently, so here goes:

YOU ARE FAT BECAUSE YOU EAT TOO MUCH OF THE WRONG STUFF, NOT BECAUSE YOU DON'T EXERCISE ENOUGH.

A study by researchers from Loyola University Health System published in the September 2008 issue of *Obesity* compares African American women in metropolitan Chicago with women in rural Nigeria. On average, the Chicago women weighed 184 pounds and the Nigerian women weighed 127 pounds. What they expected to find was that the slimmer Nigerian women would be more physically active. To their surprise, they found no significant difference between the two groups in the amount of calories burned during physical activity.

"Decreased physical activity may not be the primary driver of the obesity epidemic," states Loyola nutritionist Amy Luke, a member of the study team. "Diet is a more likely explanation than physical activity expenditure for why Chicago women weigh more than Nigerian women," Luke says. She noted that the Nigerian diet is high in fiber and carbohydrates and low in fat and animal protein. By contrast, the Chicago diet is 40-45 percent fat and high in processed foods.

A clue! Could it be better food choices?

Richard Cooper, co-author of the study and chairman of the Department of Preventive Medicine and Epidemiology dropped the bomb when he said, "We would love to say that physical activity has a positive effect on weight control, but that does not appear to be the case." Many recent studies are finding the same thing. Dr. Eric Ravussin, chair in diabetes and metabolism at Louisiana State University and exercise researcher put it more bluntly. In a Time article titled "Why Exercise Won't Make You Thin" he says, "In general, for weight loss, exercise is pretty useless." Ouch!

Deep down you already knew this, but just in case you are still in denial, the Australians were kind enough to rub our noses in it when they delivered their findings at the *2009 European Congress on Obesity*. They state "The amount of food Americans eat has been increasing since the 1970's and that alone is the cause of the obesity epidemic in the US today. Physical activity—or the lack thereof—has played virtually no role in the rising number of expanding American waistlines." Lead author Dr. Boyd Swinburn stated, "Americans have been eating more; the US Department of Agriculture data clearly show this. But US epidemiological data shows that physical activity levels haven't really changed that much. So I think we have to be much more focused on the energy-intake side of the energy-balance equation."

If it wasn't already, I think it's pretty clear what you need to do. Your focus must shift away from thinking that more time in the gym will get you where you want to be. Instead, focus on improving the quantity and quality of your diet.

It's All about the Diet

I may have given you the impression that this chapter is about eating. It's not. It's really about the relative contribution that diet and exercise make to help you get the look and feel you want. You have been lead to believe that more exercise is better if you want to lose weight; however, the focus of this book is fat loss, not weight loss.

The truth is that losing fat is 99 percent dependent upon dietary modification and one percent dependent upon exercise. That's right; for the most part, it's all about the diet. The amount of exercise you need is ridiculously small. I know this because I have observed clients in a clinical setting for many years in a row who exercise no more than 10 minutes a week. They are firm, vibrant, and look fantastic, but trust me, it's not luck. These people look this way for a reason; they work at it. Eating right is a lifestyle for them, but if you think all you need to do is change your eating habits and you will lose a bunch of fat, think again.

For fat loss both diet and exercise are essential, not optional, but do not be mislead by the small relative contribution of exercise. It plays a ***very important*** part, but it must be the right type of exercise to guarantee fat loss. Still, it's primarily all about your diet.

I've seen it happen thousands of times. Clients go through periods where they eat more or less; better or worse, and because most of my clients stick with my program for years I get to see their long-term body composition trends. On a graph showing four years worth of body composition measurements it is obvious when their eating habits improve because their body fat trends downward.

When their eating is worse their body fat trends upward. Regardless of what is happening to their fat mass, their exercise volume doesn't change.

Joe Knows Fat Loss

To illustrate the relative importance of diet and exercise I will share Joe's story with you. I had worked with Joe for many years. For the past three years he consistently weighed in around 195 pounds while averaging 67 pounds of body fat and was consistently coming in once a week for his usual ten minute high intensity exercise session.

Between the second and third quarter body composition measurements of 2007 Joe went on a popular eating plan for several weeks. His third quarter measurement revealed that he had lost 12 pounds of body weight. Twelve pounds of what, right?

As you can probably imagine, Joe was pleased with his weight loss. No matter how much I explained the absurdity of focusing on body weight to measure progress, he still wouldn't let it go. In fact, this was the same guy who walked in one day for his quarterly measurement and proceeded to strip down to his underwear. Why would he let it all hang out? So he could be as *light* as possible. My assistant and I just stood there, speechless. Old habits die hard.

For Joe to be happy with a 12 pound weight loss and stop there, he never would have known how good things really were. So I delivered the magic, "Joe, do you know why you only lost 12 pounds? It's because you gained two pounds of muscle and lost 14 pounds of fat." That is something to be very happy about because all of his weight loss was fat loss and his muscle to fat ratio shifted dramatically. He was leaner and healthier.

To sum up Joe's story, the amount of exercise he did remained constant, and because it was the right type of exercise it guaranteed fat loss. Only his eating habits changed. That's all there is to it.

Your life is about to get a lot easier and less confusing if you get one thing straight: your body will look better with good eating habits and a little bit of the right type of exercise. What is the right type of exercise? I'll give you a hint: it's not cardio.

CHAPTER EIGHT

The Right Type of Exercise

Exercise should be fun and more is better, right? Bull! This is a sure-fire way to fail. This is not the right type of exercise for you.

The fitness industry, government, doctors, and major health organizations think that more people will exercise if exercise is fun. Obviously they are wrong, because it hasn't worked so far and it never, ever will.

I would like you to experience all the benefits of exercise, the benefits that you could, and should have, but are probably missing out on. I would like to see all of you succeed at being lean, strong, and vibrant, always. But the best way to help you is not by telling you what you want to hear; it's by telling you what you need to hear. So the best way to help everyone is to vigorously promote that exercise should be very challenging, and *not* fun. So why would anyone in their right mind want to exercise? One word—success.

Believe it or not, motivation does not lead to success. Success leads to reward, which then leads to motivation. Being rewarded with great results is what motivates people to consistently exercise, not how *fun* it is. That is why you have a difficult time consistently sticking to an exercise program. Mainstream exercise recommendations simply do not reward you with great results. But that's going to change.

The right type of exercise for you is certainly not fun, but you will love how little time it takes and you will certainly love the results. In other words, you will experience success and this will keep you coming back for more. So what is the right type of exercise? High intensity strength training. In fact, it is the only form of exercise you will ever need because it is the only form of exercise capable of providing you with every exercise-related health and fitness benefit known to man at this point in time. It is so effective that it renders all other forms of exercise obsolete and optional.

Brenda's Fountain of Youth

Brenda is 56 and has worked under my guidance for the past eight years. What has her exercise program consisted of for the past eight years? One very brief and challenging strength training workout each week. Does she look forward to her workout each week? Hell no. It's hard work. It's uncomfortable. So why does she keep doing it week after week, year after year, and paying me no less? "It's addicting," Brenda says. The truth is it works better than the hours of free weight classes and five mile runs she used to do several times a week. She feels the difference. She sees the difference, and so does everyone else. Over the past four years her body fat percentage has trended downward while her lean body mass has trended upward. Her arms and thighs are rock hard and she has a physical capacity greater than most young men. Eight years from now she will be doing the same exercise program, still be in great shape, and getting further ahead while others fall further behind.

Are you getting better with age?

Even though *chronologically* Brenda is getting older, *metabolically* she is getting younger. In fact, the body composition scale I use has a feature we all like to watch just for fun. It's called *metabolic age*. When I started measuring Brenda four years ago, she was 52 with a metabolic age of 50. Now at 56 she has a metabolic age of 42. The gap between her chronological age and metabolic age keeps getting wider as time marches on. This will happen when your muscles get stronger and you lose fat.

The Free Time Factor

You may be thinking, "I've never stuck with any exercise program that long." Besides great results, do you know what makes it even easier for Brenda to stick with it? Over the last eight years she has averaged 44 workouts per year. Her average workout time is between six and eight minutes each week and her total exercise time annually is just under six hours. That's right – *six hours a year*. Yes, she spends less time exercising in one year than many people spend in two weeks. And her results are better *because of this*. But I know what you're thinking, and trust me, Brenda does too. Many people have asked Brenda what she does to stay in such good shape and when she tells them what she does the response is "That's impossible!" So why would you think this way?

In my opinion you react this way because of conditioned thinking. You have been told for years that you must exercise for at least 30 to 60 minutes. You also know that you cannot exert yourself very hard to keep a pace that will allow you to last this long. So when someone says they only workout for less than 10 minutes a week, you filter that number through the context of what your own workout is like – not very intense and probably not giving you the results you expect. So you think, "How could fewer minutes work better? That's impossible!" But you would be wrong.

The Most Costly Exercise Mistakes

What makes it possible for Brenda to achieve such good results with such a brief workout? I make sure she avoids the three most costly exercise mistakes – *too easy*, *too much*, and *too often*.

The key here is *intensity*. That is what you must consider when you read "six minute workout." Brenda's exercise is very intense; it's no walk in the park, but you should know that anyone can do it, no matter his or her age or physical condition. In fact, I have watched frail 90 year-old men and women train with great intensity and regain a physical capacity they had lost 20 years ago. Still, the only way to understand high intensity exercise is to experience it first hand, but I will do my best to describe it so you can get a sense of what it's all about.

I use the following example because I think the chin-up is the easiest exercise for most people to picture in their minds. It doesn't matter if you can actually do a chin-up; just allow your imagination to play along for the sake of explanation.

Imagine standing on a chair and placing your chin above a chin up bar. As you slowly bend your knees and lift both feet off the chair you pull up hard with both arms, attempting to prevent your body from descending. Your goal is to keep your body up in the same position as long as you can; this could be anywhere from one to forty-five seconds. Once your muscles fatigue to a point where you can no longer maintain your starting position, despite your very best effort to prevent downward movement, you are finished. It's that simple. Move on to your next exercise.

What goes up must come down. This is true if you are using your own body weight or the weight stack on an exercise machine at the gym. In the example above your body wants to go in one direction, and you want it to go in another. As each second passes your muscles shake and burn, but you keep pulling. You breathe heavily and get warmer, but keep on pulling. You want to stop because it is uncomfortable, but keep pulling. Within seconds your muscles will be so tired that there will be no way you can prevent your body from descending. This is called maximum effort. This is the first requirement for getting the look you want, and you should strive to thoroughly exhaust your muscles during each exercise you do every time you workout. The exhaustion should occur in no more than 45 seconds. If you can go on longer than this you don't have enough resistance and the exercise is too easy. Don't make that mistake.

So what does this mean? Contrary to what you have been lead to believe, you do not suffer from a lack of movement. You suffer from lack of significant *resistance* to your movement. Get the resistance correct and you will never again entertain the thought of doing low intensity activities to get in shape.

It Should Never Get Easier

This brings us to another question I am frequently asked, "Brian, will this ever get any easier?" The answer is no! I make it perfectly clear during consultations that it should never get easier and if it ever does then we are doing something wrong.

Brenda has been exercising consistently for eight years, and her progress now comes at a slow pace, but at each workout I always add resistance, even if it's a small one-eighth of a pound washer. At each workout it should be your goal to add more resistance, no matter how little it may be. Always strive to "inch the ball forward." The higher the resistance progresses, the younger you stay.

What should get easier for you? Everything else you do in your life—lifting grandchildren, yard work, travel, recreational activities, and anything else that involves movement.

Remember, the strength of your muscles determines the state of your entire physiology. If you are not getting stronger you are getting weaker. If you are getting weaker you are aging much faster than you should, and probably getting fatter too. To keep your muscle to fat ratio *young* you must regularly (once every seven to ten days) challenge your muscles intensely. If you dial back your effort, your body will return to the comfort of deterioration. There is no such thing as maintenance. Maintenance will surely lead to regression.

Checks and Balances

Once you get your intensity level correct, it becomes much easier to avoid the other two costly exercise mistakes—*too much* and *too often*.

Let's get back to Brenda. She is very strong. I position her on the leg press exercise with her knees extended into a 130-degree bend as she resists the downward movement of 640 pounds. After 45 seconds of resisting the descent of the weight every muscle in her legs is completely spent and unable to resist any longer, so the weight descends despite her best effort to stop it. Not bad for a woman with a body weight of 138 pounds, right?

The point is, when the resistance is correct your maximum strength capacity will be challenged and it will be physically impossible for you to last long before your muscles are thoroughly exhausted. There is a built in check and balance. The higher the resistance, the lower the time of exertion. Your body protects itself from doing too much. This is why Brenda's workouts are so short. But do not be mislead by the brevity. Could Brenda tolerate more minutes of such intensity? She probably could, but would it be necessary? No. Those 45 seconds of all out effort are like flipping on a light switch in her leg muscles. Once the light is on you don't have to keep pushing upward on the switch; the light is already on and it isn't going to get any brighter. One intense burst is enough. To stop, rest, and do the same exercise again would simply be wasted effort for no productive purpose. She simply moves to her next exercise and repeats the same procedure until she has completed three or four exercises. Her workout for the week is then complete.

Regular Exercise

What does Brenda do after her workout? She goes on living her life and waiting for seven days before she does it again. Why so long? I won't let her do it more frequently. Working out too often will actually prevent her muscles and all the systems that support and supply her muscles from fully recovering prior to her next workout. If her body does not fully recover, she will gradually become weaker and never get the benefits she wants.

The question going through your head right now is probably, "If she doesn't work out for seven days won't she get worse?" Absolutely not. Remember, her workout is the means to the end, not the end itself. Her workout stimulated her body to change. Now it is up to her body to make those changes. This takes time and rest. During those seven days off Brenda's body is *recovering* from intense exertion. It is rebuilding back to its pre-workout condition and then *supercompensating*, or upgrading its capability to a new and improved level. How can she get worse when this is happening? She can't. There is only one way for her to go— up! Brenda actually rests her way to success. Cool concept, right?

A few years ago one of my clients was forced to take four weeks off from exercise due to a family emergency. Even though this was a stressful time filled with travel and pressure, the break from exercise and time to sleep more certainly did not hurt. Upon her return from one month without exercise I decided to check her body composition. Cindy had gained five pounds—of what you ask? Her lean body mass increased eight pounds while her fat mass *decreased* by three pounds. She was leaner. She felt rested and looked rested. As a result her workout was stellar. I gave her more resistance and she either matched, or exceeded her performance times from four weeks earlier. See what extra rest can do for you? By the way, I see this happen to clients *all the time*. It is no fluke. Most people are so stressed and tired that they never realize their true potential for fat loss and muscle gain.

Trust me, the right type of exercise means never having to exercise all the time. Your exercise should only be as regular as it takes your body to fully recover from your last workout. For most people that will be approximately seven days.

The scientist in me is always pushing to find out how little exercise people need to get great results. I am not searching to see how much exercise people can tolerate. That doesn't make any sense, and besides, I have already tried that and it simply doesn't work. One thing I can guarantee you is that you will always have the best changes in your muscle to fat ratio with harder, briefer, and less frequent exercise. This combination will beat any other exercise recommendation hands down every time.

The Cornerstone of Vitality

At this point you may be thinking, "Is he saying that I shouldn't do any other type of activity?" Absolutely not. Over the years I have had many people enter my program who are already very active. Many of them regularly participate in yoga, jogging, tennis, spinning, and various other types of activities several days a week. When they add high intensity strength training to their mix of weekly activities, their performance in ALL of those activities is improved, and their bodies develop firmness like never before. I frequently listen to stories about changing body shape, improved energy level, and ease of movement. In fact, they often develop a strong desire to be even more active.

On the other hand, I have seen many of the same people decrease, or totally eliminate their various activities *except* strength training and continue to enjoy a level of physical fitness greater than they had before they started the program and became stronger. Why?

Strong muscles are the cornerstone of youthful vitality, and being active is a natural by-product of having strong muscles. But simply being active does not give you strong muscles. Therefore, as long as high intensity strength training is part of your life, extra activity becomes something you *choose* to do, not something you *have* to do. For example, if one weekend you play three sets of tennis on Saturday and go for a 15 mile hike on Sunday and the next weekend you feel like lying on the couch reading a book, great! As long as strength training is a constant in your life, and you continuously strive to become stronger, your physical fitness will be excellent and you will enjoy a firm and leaner body. This is one of the perks that makes it much easier for my clients to stick with their strength training program for so long; it means freedom from the pressure that you have to exercise all the time to be in good shape. They have learned that it simply isn't true and see no reason to go back to doing things the "old way." This has important implications for your fat loss.

I believe there are many people sitting on the sidelines because they think getting in shape requires a lot of time spent exercising. It's simply not true! As I have already stated, more exercise is actually a great way to kill fat loss and promote fat gain. You may be one of those people on the sidelines, or someone who wishes there was a less time-consuming option. Whoever you are, knowing that you only need one form of exercise, and that anything beyond that is optional can be a huge stress relief. This makes losing fat, gaining muscle, and reshaping your body much more efficient and enjoyable.

The Fun Part

If exercise should not be fun, where is the fun part? It's fun when someone underestimates your age by 10 years! It's fun when you can lift a 50-pound bag of potting soil by yourself and not hurt your back. It's fun when you feel great all the time. It's fun when you notice a head turn to look at your attractive body. The benefits are endless, and I could go on and on and tell you thousands of stories from people who have lived a better quality of life because they are willing to be a little uncomfortable for just a few minutes a week.

Wouldn't you like to be one of those stories?

Think differently. If you want to look and feel your best make high intensity strength training the cornerstone of your fitness regimen. You have no idea how much better your life will be because of it.

CHAPTER NINE

Exercise in Futility

In order to get what you want—a more attractive body—you must first get what you need: more muscle and less fat. In the previous chapter I talked about the most effective form of exercise for making this happen for you, and you may have reacted with disbelief. "But don't you still need cardio?" you ask. No, you don't. Cardio won't even get you close to what you need. In fact, it will get you what you don't want and make things much worse. But you don't believe me, so off you go for one of your wonderful cardio workouts.

At this point you have learned that your workout won't burn very many extra calories, at least not enough to make it worth the hour of your free time you devote to burning them. As a result of the extra activity your appetite will increase and you will want to eat more, which will make it difficult to stay on your latest diet. And because you do the same jog at the same pace your movement becomes increasingly more efficient which means you actually burn fewer and fewer calories each time you work out. It's really sort of funny, but all your calorie-burning efforts are taking you in the wrong direction. But you don't believe me, so on you go, and it gets even worse.

Do you know why you can keep going for one hour? Your exercise is way too easy. Rather than challenging a large percentage of all your muscle fibers and the maximum strength they possess, you are engaging a very small percentage of your smallest and weakest muscle fibers over and over again. So your largest and strongest muscle fibers—the fibers that will have a dramatic, positive effect on your appearance and health—are considered baggage. They atrophy and fade away, never to be heard from again. You will regret this 20 years from now when you fall and break a hip.

Remember, you need more muscle, not less, but that's exactly what you are going to get. Mother Nature has a rule: if you don't use it, you lose it. So as the muscle fibers that say "Look at me, I'm firm and fit" wither, so does your resting metabolic rate, energy level, and youthful shape.

Muscle is active tissue. It uses energy to stay alive. As you plod along week after week, in a year's time you can lose one pound of that energy-consuming muscle. This may reduce your daily energy expenditure by a dozen calories. Although it doesn't sound like much, this small increase in the gap between your daily energy intake and energy expenditure will lead to big increases in body fat over time. This means the loss of muscle is going to make it next to impossible for you to keep fat off your body no matter how little you eat. Sound familiar?

By the way, just in case you think you are going to get a post-workout-calorie-burning-boost from easy exercise, think again. Mother Nature doesn't like to expend energy unnecessarily, so after your workout your body will reset to its pre-exercise resting metabolic rate quickly. Unfortunately, as time marches on and your muscle mass dwindles your reset point becomes lower and lower. Your fat cells love this. But you don't believe me, so on you go.

Your knees ache. Your shins hurt. Your back is killing you. Now you add injury to insult. The one thing that your exercise can do very well is produce injury. How can it not? It's repetitive. It's forceful. It's frequent. And please do not feed me the "But it's low impact" load of crap. There does not have to be *impact* for your joints to experience force and for injury to occur. Just ask a baseball pitcher if his shoulder surgeries were the result of his arm *hitting* something. I constantly consult with many people who have had to stop using their elliptical machine or recumbent bike—two supposedly "low impact" devices—due to achy knees. Just burn those things.

Excess fat is your enemy, not your knees, hips, and back. In a 2007 *New York Times* article titled "Whatever Happened to Jane Fonda in Tights?" jewelry designer Olivia Siemens complains that "Swimming is just about the only exercise I can do these days. I'm a fashion victim—the fashion of aerobics." She recalls taking as many as six aerobics classes a week in the 80's. "It was supposedly all about staying in shape but look at me: I can hardly walk."

Cardio should come with a warning label—it is guaranteed injury. It will cripple you eventually. So if you think losing weight is difficult now, think how hard it is going to be when your joints can't tolerate much of *any* activity. But it can't happen to you, so you pop a few Advil and on you go.

Everyone thinks that exercise is a great way to lose fat. What everyone doesn't know is that exercise is a lousy way to lose fat. To understand why, you must consider what you are doing to your body in the context of biology. In their book *Lights Out*, authors T.S Wiley and Bent Formby provide a perfect explanation:

Note: Prior to reading the following quote you need to be familiar with the term *cortisol*. Cortisol is a stress hormone involved in the response to stress and anxiety. Among its many functions, cortisol accelerates the breakdown of body proteins, increases blood glucose levels, and weakens the activity of the immune system.

"*When you exercise day and night to stave off the weight gain your body and mind crave, you kick in your 'stress response.' The message you're sending to your systems is 'Oh, my God, a famine's coming and there's a tiger chasing me!!'*

"*Trust us, this is no solution.*

"*In fact, exercise just might be the last nail in our collective coffins. The stress response enacted when you run for your life on that treadmill causes your cortisol levels to rise.*

If you do this once in a while, say, every ten days, the natural episodic cortisol response will keep your heart and brain healthy. But if you exercise like a maniac more than once a week, the high cortisol levels resulting from all of the chronic exercise actually mimics the stress of mating season, when the long hours of light and the competition (especially for males) kept cortisol at yearly highs.

"*In this chronic state, not only are you keeping your blood sugar up, taxing your insulin response system with cortisol's blood-sugar-mobilizing effects, you are actually becoming insulin-resistant as you exercise, too. This fact means exercise can make you fat.*"

I thought you wanted less fat?

At this point, let's review how cardio is "helping" you. You can think of a million things you would rather be doing with your time, things that would be much more enjoyable and productive. You really aren't burning as many extra calories as you think, and burning fewer and fewer each time because your movement is more efficient. You are working up a ravenous appetite which will not only drive you to eat more and completely erase all the calories you have burned, but will make it much harder to stay on your diet. You are probably grumpy. Your resting metabolism is slowly declining because your muscles are getting weaker and the jiggle in your thighs isn't firming up. And the worst part is the stress your body feels makes it store what little food you do eat as fat. No wonder someone occasionally asks if you are feeling all right. You probably look tired, pale, and much older than you really are. That doesn't sound like help to me. With friends like cardio who needs enemies? But you can't stop. You are an addict. You need your fix, so on you go.

Many years ago I was working with two clients, one was a retired endocrinologist, and the other was a running addict with osteoporosis in both feet and a stress fracture in one. Although she cut back significantly, she continued to run. I couldn't understand why. What was driving so many people to continue to do activity that was obviously destroying their body?

I began questioning the doctor about exercise addiction. Was it real? He told me that it was very real and that anyone trying to "come off" exercise would exhibit some of the same basic symptoms as someone coming off heroin or any other addictive substance.

My experience was consistent with his assertion. I had a new business pioneering a radically new way to exercise—no cardio and only a brief high intensity strength training workout once a week—and on several occasions when I asked clients to give up constant cardio to improve their results, not many could do it, even if they wanted to.

In a 2002 *New York Times* article titled "Runner's High? Endorphins? Fiction, Some Scientists Say," Dr. Virginia Grant, a psychologist at the Memorial University of Newfoundland studied exercise and addiction in rats. She found that rats allowed to run seemed unable to stop. Could this behavior be similar to rats addicted to cocaine or morphine? The answer appears to be yes.

Rats like to nibble all day long, but in this experiment the rats were offered food for only one hour a day. "Animals that were left in their cages, without running wheels and without food for the other 23 hours did fine; they quickly learned to eat all their day's calories in one hour long session. But those that had running wheels for those 23 hours ran so much that they could not eat enough to compensate, actually eating less and less as they ran more and more reaching distances of 12 miles by running nonstop. In a week or two, nearly all were dead of starvation."

You may be doing the same thing—using exercise as a distraction, or your drug of choice. Too bad no one is passing food through your door. You can find more than enough to compensate.

What made running irresistible for these rats? A growing body of science is finding that many addictions are the same; they share a common pathway within the brain with a common chemical signal: a flood of the nerve hormone dopamine.

"A reward is something you work for," says Dr. Roy Wise, an addiction researcher at the National Institute of Drug Abuse. "It makes you want to go back for more. It's a positive feedback in the brain that keeps saying, yes, yes,

yes. That's what the dopamine system is for. The bottom line is that you will like anything you can do that turns on these dopamine neurons." Just like cardio.

Why do we even have a pathway like this? As you huff and puff, the blood volume going to your brain decreases from 13 percent at rest to 8 percent during light exercise to 4 percent during heavy exercise. The lack of oxygen to your brain triggers neural bursts that many scientists believe may account for near-death experiences of euphoria and tranquility. The same area of the brain also becomes electrically active when a person thinks about God or spirituality. Could this be why running has been described by many as a religious experience?

Again, I return to *Lights Out* for proper biological context:

"The truth is all that exercise is doing more than making you high. It's exacerbating the burnout of your cortisol receptors. Running is a fear response. In the real world, it means something is after you; at least that's what your body and brain thinks. If you run long enough, all your systems believe you're not going to outrun that predator. The brain chemistry that follows extended running has evolved to make your exit from this world more pleasant. This means that oxygen depletion alone will kick in the part of the brain that takes you to heaven or, in this world, gives you a reason to keep running. The mechanism of brain chemistry that causes you to see God as you run out of oxygen evolved from programmed

responses—responses to environmental cues that no longer exist, responses that once upon a time might have kept you alive or made dying okay. Now, they're killing you."

If you can't stop the cardio, you may be a junkie, and by the way, you're also destroying your body.

At the beginning of this chapter I told you that in order to get what you want you must first get what you need. What do you want? An attractive body... ASAP. What do you need to make this happen? More muscle and less fat, but the best way to make this happen is by getting stronger and *reducing* the amount of stress your body feels. Cardio does just the opposite.

Someone has to say it and I am more than happy to be the one. If everyone stopped doing cardio right now the collective health of our nation would rise exponentially overnight, guaranteed. Hire a shrink, check yourself into rehab, or go cold turkey, but whatever you do, stop wasting your time with cardio. The more you embrace cardio the further away from a healthy and attractive body you get.

CHAPTER TEN

You Can't Make Your Heart Stronger

Whenever I tell someone about the futility of cardio, they usually respond, "What about my heart?" I say, what about it? Do you think your heart can tell if you are walking, jogging, or lifting and lowering weights? Of course not. All it knows is that it must supply blood to working muscles. Makes sense, right? And yet I hear it all the time, "But the heart is a muscle. You need cardio to keep the heart muscle strong." This reminds me of the words of Anatole France:

If fifty million people say a foolish thing it is still a foolish thing.

The notion that you can make your heart stronger or healthier through exercise is completely false! If this is your reason for doing all that walking and jogging, STOP! You are wasting your time, wasting your muscles, and making yourself fatter.

It's true; the heart is a muscle—*a cardiac muscle*. Cardiac muscle is *involuntary*, meaning you have no willful control over its function. Skeletal muscle, like those in your arms and legs, is voluntary. You willfully control when to relax, when to contract, and with how much force. But don't take my word for it. The following quote is right out of Arthur

C. Guyton's *Textbook of Medical Physiology*:

> *The two basic means by which the volume pumped by the heart is regulated are (1) intrinsic autoregulation of pumping in response to changes in volume of blood flowing into the heart and (2) reflex control of the heart by the autonomic nervous system.*

Intrinsic autoregulation? Reflex control? Just in case you missed it, notice the prefix *auto* in the words *autonomic* and *autoregulation*? That means *self*. The body does it on its own.

Now, I'm no cardiologist, but it sure sounds to me like it's out of our control.

You have a resting cardiac output of approximately five liters of blood per minute. Depending on what you are doing from second to second, and without additional help from your nervous system, heart rate and strength of contraction can be adjusted automatically to provide a cardiac output up to 15 liters of blood per minute. This is the *normal* physiological capability of your heart. Exercise has no effect on this capability; you are born with it. Should you need a turbo boost beyond your normal capability, sympathetic nerves can increase the pumping ability of your heart to as high as 25 liters of blood per minute. Again, you are born with this capability and it occurs automatically.

To give this more perspective for you, a cardiac output of 15 liters of blood per minute would roughly equate to a heart rate of approximately 130 beats per minute. A cardiac output of 25 liters of blood per minute would equate to a heart rate of approximately 200 beats per minute.

So off you go for your jog because it keeps your heart strong and healthy. For this to happen you would need to be challenging your heart beyond its capability, after all, this is how you make muscles stronger, and the heart is a muscle, right? Let's see how it goes.

Most of you out there don't know, or even care about your heart rate while you exercise. Good! Like your body weight, it leads you in the wrong direction. You just do what you are told—complete your 60 minutes a few times a week.

Let's assume you are 45 years old with a resting heart rate of 65 beats per minute. Not only are you concerned about your heart, but you also want to exercise in your "fat burning zone" so you want to keep your heart rate steady on the lower end of the zone for best results. According to the Karvonen Target Heart Rate Formula that would mean your target heart rate would be 137 beats per minute. And off you go with your heart beating 137 times each minute for 60 minutes.

Was this challenging for your heart? Well, without much effort it was capable of automatically pumping 15 liters of blood per minute. At your pace that was nearly all you needed. Even if you felt like turning on the jets to sprint for 60 yards and made your heart rate soar to 200 beats per minute your heart would automatically adjust and pump out 25 liters of blood per minute. So did you challenge your heart's capability in any way? No. And keep in mind that the typical person doing their cardio moves at a pace far below that cited in this example.

It should now be perfectly clear to you that your heart is an *involuntary* organ that can adapt itself from second-to-second to just about any demand you throw at it. It can pump as little as 2-3 liters of blood per minute all the way up to 25 liters of blood per minute. It can change its own rate of pumping and strength of contraction automatically. In other words, exercise cannot give your heart a capability that it doesn't already have. Exercise will not make your heart *stronger*.

It's Your Muscles Knucklehead

Does cardio really condition the cardiovascular system? Consider the following quotes:

> *When patients participate in exercise programs, they often assume that their heart becomes stronger. This is not the case. Physical training results in a sense of well being because of other effects… it improves the efficiency of the muscles…it improves the hormonal tone of the body…it improves the control of sugar in people with diabetes. However, exercise will not make the heart beat more strongly.*
>
> *Bruce D. Charash, MD, Cardiologist – From his book, Heart Myths, 1991*

> *You might suspect from the emphasis on cardiopulmonary fit-*

ness that the major effect of training is on the heart and lungs. Guess again. Exercise does nothing for the lungs that has been amply proved...nor does it especially benefit your heart. Running, no matter what you have been told, primarily trains and conditions the muscles.

George Sheehan, MD, Cardiologist – A 1981 article in The Physician and Sports Medicine.

Most of the improvement in functional capacity due to exercise is not even directly related to the heart. It is due to an effect on the peripheral muscle cells whereby they more efficiently extract oxygen from the blood.

Henry Solomon, MD, Cardiologist – From his book, The Exercise Myth, 1987

Did you notice the common denominator in each quote? It's *muscle.*

Cardio simply makes your muscles a little stronger, which gives the illusion that your heart and lungs are stronger. It is the improvement in muscular strength that makes you feel like you are improving and getting in shape.

A 1996 study in the *Journal of Cardiopulmonary Rehabilitation* perfectly illustrates this concept. Women ages 60-77 performed a weight-loaded and non weight-loaded graded walking test on a treadmill. The weight-loaded test required that the women walk at two miles per hour while holding a box weighing 40 percent of their maximum biceps strength, while the non weight-loaded test required a normal walk at two miles per hour. Both tests were performed before and after sixteen weeks of a workout consisting solely of weight training three times per week. At the end of the sixteen-week training period, total body strength had increased by 57 percent. The results of both follow-up treadmill tests showed reduced heart rate (the subjects weren't breathing as hard), reduced systolic blood pressure (the heart didn't need to pump as hard), and reduced rate-pressure product (the heart needed less oxygen to perform the same task).

The authors concluded that weight training *reduces* cardiovascular stress.

Did the women in this study improve their heart and lung function? No. So how could these results happen if they didn't do cardio? The answer is simple—their muscles became stronger. To further explain, let's say that before the weight training program began, ten muscle fibers were required to complete the treadmill test. After the weight training program, when muscle strength was improved, five muscle fibers were capable of performing the same task that previously required ten. Therefore, the cardiovascular system only needed to work half as hard to do the same work. Makes sense, doesn't it?

Just remember, the reason exercise is important is not because of the effect it has on your heart, but because of the effect it has on your muscles. Stronger muscles are more efficient. They extract oxygen and get rid of waste products more efficiently. Weak muscles are inefficient. Weak muscles put more stress on your heart. Why would you want to do that? Does your car function better as you put more miles on it?

Neil Armstrong once said, "I believe that every human has a finite number of heartbeats. I don't intend to waste any of mine running around doing exercises." Learn from Neil. I want to save your heart, so it's time for you to think differently about the relationship between your exercise and your heart. Rather than wasting heartbeats and placing more stress on your heart with exercise, your goal should be to make your muscles as strong as possible for the purpose of placing less stress on your heart. Doesn't that make more sense? This is what I call *real* cardiovascular benefit.

You have nothing to worry about. Your heart is just fine.

CHAPTER ELEVEN

Real Health Insurance

Here's how it goes for all you "weight-watchers" out there: you diet without the right type of exercise and lose muscle mass. You reach your goal and get comfortable, or get frustrated because you can't get those last five pounds off, and then you go off your diet and start eating like you used to. What happens?

It's the weight loss/fat gain rollercoaster. Notice I didn't say weight loss/weight gain rollercoaster. If only you were that lucky to *just* gain back the weight of the water and muscle mass you lost. But it doesn't work that way. You gain back all fat. So you continue on this ride throughout your lifetime going up and down and getting fatter and fatter. Why?

When you lose muscle mass your resting metabolism declines. This means your body burns fewer calories at rest. This makes it next to impossible to keep your fat cells from thriving and calling the shots.

You can get off this ride any time you want.

Wouldn't it be nice to get the fat off and keep if off forever? Wouldn't it be nice if you had some kind of assurance that you would never have to ride the rollercoaster again?

Of course it would, and you can do it if you do one simple thing—get stronger.

I've said it before and I'll say it again: high intensity strength training is essential if you want a shot at keeping fat off forever. It is the most misunderstood secret weapon against a fat body. It is real health insurance.

I see the protective effect of strong muscles all the time when clients go on vacation. They eat and they drink, usually much more than normal, but hey, they have a good time and that is what you do on vacation. When they come back the first thing I hear about is how fat they feel. But are they really fatter? I like to know, so after they stop protesting, I finally get them to step on the body composition monitor.

Why do they initially not want to check their body composition? Because they know they are heavier. Big deal. Yes, despite my incessant reminding, they are still terrorized by their weight. But I know what is about to happen. They don't gain any body fat. In fact, I often see their fat mass decrease and their lean body mass increase, even though their weight goes up! They can't believe it. It's amazing what rest and relaxation can do for your body composition. So what's going on here?

Well, there are a couple things. Strength training can help you reclaim lost muscle mass. In fact, it is not uncommon to see a three-pound increase after just three months of strength training. Also, the resting metabolic rate of stronger muscles is higher, and that means a higher fluid content.

Dr. Wayne Wescott, fitness researcher and senior fitness executive at the South Shore YMCA in Quincy, Massachusetts, suggests that strength training may increase the resting metabolic rate of muscle by 1.5 calories per pound per day. He uses the example of a 155-pound man with a resting metabolic rate of 1600 calories per day with approximately 62 pounds of skeletal muscle. If each pound uses 5.7 calories per day at rest, the contribution to his resting metabolism is about 353 calories. If he adds three pounds of muscle, and each pound of stronger muscle now uses 7.2 calories per day at rest, then the new contribution to this resting metabolism is about 468 calories. Now he expends an additional 115 calories each day. This is about a seven percent increase in his resting metabolism.

The same thing can happen for you when you get stronger. This is your wiggle room. This is your insurance, and it's permanent as long as you keep striving to get stronger.

In a *HealthDay News* article titled "Lifting Weights Keeps Overweight at Bay," a study conducted by Kathryn Schmitz, an assistant professor at the University of Pennsylvania's Center for Clinical Epidemiology and Biostatistics shows how valuable strong muscles can be. Her study included 164 overweight (overfat and undermuscled) and obese women ages 24 to 44 who were divided into two groups. One group participated in a 16 week supervised strength training program that was followed up with four "booster" workouts per year for the next two years. The other group received a brochure that recommended they get 30 minutes to an hour of aerobic exercise most days of the week. Both groups were told not to change their diets in any way that might lead to body weight changes, which I'm sure they were happy to hear.

At the end of the two-year period the women in the strength training group showed an average 3.7 percent decrease in body fat while the women in the aerobics group showed no change in body fat. That shouldn't surprise you after everything you have learned to this point. Nevertheless, for a 180 pound woman with 30 percent body fat this could mean a 10 pound decrease in body fat. If someone said you could be two years older and 10 pounds leaner would you want that? Of course you would.

Although I don't advocate that you regularly overeat to test your coverage, if you do so on occasion, strong muscles are always there to protect you from gaining fat. Now science is beginning to uncover much more. You are in better hands than originally thought.

The science of *epigenetics* is discovering that based on your lifestyle choices, particularly diet and exercise, you can alter how your DNA is expressed. In other words, you can alter your genetic fingerprint to favor leanness or fatness on the fly throughout your lifetime. It's never too late to make this change.

It's seems reasonable to think that all of the tissues in your body cooperate with each other for your benefit. However, epigenetics is finding that different body tissues compete for building blocks to increase their presence and further their own agenda. Eat a poor diet that promotes a fat body and you will turn on genetic switches that will help your fat cells compete more efficiently for your body's resources. Or stress your muscles with high intensity exercise and you will flip a switch that allows your muscles a greater competitive advantage.

Even more amazing is that flipping these genetic switches will even alter your behavior. Yes, the way you act and think will change to ensure that a particular body tissue maintains a competitive advantage. No, it's not something you are aware of. It just happens.

I observed this frequently with clients who did not want to change their poor dietary habits to improve their physical transformation results. After learning that there was no point in talking to someone about change if they didn't want to change, I quit talking about diet. Then I noticed an interesting pattern develop.

After a few months had passed clients were stronger and more energetic. Their bodies were firmer and they were generally feeling good about themselves. Out of nowhere they would begin to ask questions about dietary changes. They were thinking about healthier options. I hadn't prompted it. So where was this coming from? I think their muscles were now calling the shots. Their muscles were now competing for a bigger piece of the action. They wanted to thrive, and any behavior that contributed to a healthier body would further their agenda.

Who do you want to win, your fat cells or your muscle cells? I know; it's a dumb question. So change the odds in favor of your muscles. By taking just one simple step—starting a high intensity strength training program—you will put yourself in a position to lose fat and keep fat off your body forever. By simply getting stronger you can unleash a host of behaviors that tip the balance in favor of a lean and vibrant body. You will be on autopilot so more muscle and less fat comes naturally for you. Now that's insurance worth investing in.

CHAPTER TWELVE

Religion, Sex, Politics, and...Diet

There is an old saying I have found useful for surviving in the business world: Never talk about religion, sex, or politics. They are very personal subjects and can lead to big problems if your views don't match those of your audience.

In my line of work the first question often asked is "How soon can I see results?" My response to this is "How soon are you willing to change the way you eat?" These are fightin' words to a lot of people. Why? Because most people know they don't eat well, but they don't want anyone pointing it out to them. It's personal. So after many years of wasting my time talking about dietary choices and offending many clients, I revised the old saying to "Never talk about religion, sex, politics, or *diet*." Most people are set in their ways and don't want to change. Until they are ready to change there is no point in talking about food choices.

Now I bristle anytime the subject comes up. It's not that I don't want to talk about better dietary choices; I certainly do because I want to help people get where they want to go. The questions "How should I eat?" or "What should I eat?" bother me because I don't think I should need to answer these for anyone. You already know what you should eat. There really isn't much to say. I simply do not believe that you don't know that eating naturally grown fresh fruits and vegetables is better than eating a bunch of heavily processed, chemical-laden foods. Just go and do it.

If you were hoping to find a structured menu plan complete with recipes in this book you're going to be disappointed. This is not another diet plan book. While recipes and menus would give you something concrete to follow on your way to a better body, they aren't necessary. All you need is trust in your own internal wisdom. This is what will free you from the grip of brilliant food marketing and allow you to gain back control of your life. Although on one level you already know what you should eat, that's not the level you operate on, so I would rather discuss a few things that contribute to shaping the way you think, which consequently keep you fat.

In his book *The Omnivores Dilemma: A Natural History of Four Meals*, author Michael Pollan states that "how you feel about eating may be just as important as what you eat." I contend that most people don't have any thoughts or feelings about eating. They just do it. They are unconscious with respect to what they put in their bodies and why. That's where the problem lies.

The User Illusion

I remember a colleague once saying that people will spend a million dollars on a bona fide lie but won't spend five bucks on the truth. Care to guess why the weight loss industry is a billion dollar a year success? It isn't because it sells a solution that actually works. It sells a fantasy—you can have what you want without any effort or change in your lifestyle. That's a lie.

You are being used.

It's called The User Illusion. You, as the user of your life, have the illusion that you are in control of most decisions you make, including food choices. Trust me on this; you are definitely not in control, at least not consciously. But you could be.

Identity Therapist Dr. Lynn Seiser explains. "Everywhere you look a subliminal message is coming at you, but you cannot pay attention to everything. And because there are no filters on your sensory inputs—sight, sound, and feelings—everything that happens around you is registered with some strength whether you are aware of it or not. It's the stuff you are not aware of that actually controls you. Why? Because there is more of it and you don't know it's there."

There is a communication theory about the magic number seven plus or minus two. We can consciously pay attention to a certain amount of stimulus. At five pieces of information there is not enough to entertain our conscious mind and out of boredom, we turn off. At nine pieces of information there is too much for our conscious to entertain and we turn off. The problem is the information just keeps coming.

So, before you actually know what you think, how you feel, or act, when you make a food choice all the unconscious subliminal messages and preconditioned patterns control what you do. You don't make a conscious decision, hence, the illusion of control.

One thing I have noticed about people is that they have become spectators in their lives. They are not mindful of most things that occur in their lives, especially food choices. They don't read labels. They don't ask questions. They don't investigate what is really good for them. If it's convenient and tastes good it goes in the mouth. They are on autopilot with no direction.

The good news is that all the unconscious messages and programs only work if you are not aware of them. Being mindful of what you are doing gets you off autopilot. Being aware of what you are doing allows you to see through the unconscious programming and take charge of making good food choices. Rather than reacting to unconscious unknown external messages, you respond from your own internal sense of wisdom.

Trust yourself, not others to make a decision for you. The answers are within you. All you have to do is let yourself find them. For example, if you eat something and don't feel well after, that's a good indication that it's something you shouldn't be eating, so don't eat it again. Is that hard? All you have to do is start paying attention and see through the illusions.

Be the user of your life, not the one being used.

Crabs in a Bucket

It seems like you're damned if you do and damned if you don't. Becoming more conscious of how you eat will most likely not be as hard for you as it is for others around you.

It's Crab Bucket Syndrome. When a single crab is put into a lidless bucket, it can and will escape. However, when more than one crab share a bucket, none can get out. If one crab elevates himself above the others, they will grab him and drag him back down to share the mutual fate of the rest of the group—going nowhere. Crab bucket syndrome is often used to describe situations where one person is attempting to better himself and others in the community attempt to pull him back down. Misery loves company, right?

If you are going to take steps to improve yourself through better dietary choices, be prepared to take some heat. You are going to make other people uncomfortable and they will do their best to drag you down so they feel better.

I see Crab Bucket Syndrome all the time, especially when a client makes better dietary choices. I listened on several occasions as Katy told me what others were saying to her while she was going through my fat loss program. She got to experience how others really feel about themselves.

Katy is determined and when she makes up her mind that she is going to do something she does it all the way. For six weeks Katy was going to follow a structured menu and rest plan. To reduce the stress of making such a change, Katy wanted to remove herself from the temptations associated with certain social situations. "One of my friends actually lectured me about what I was doing because it prevented me from going out with her," Katy said. She heard "Why are you doing that? That isn't good for you," and "I would never do that." "It happened several times," Katy said. "My friends just said call me when you're finished with that stupid diet."

The good news is that despite all of the grabbing and pulling, the crabs did not keep Katy down. She went on to lose 10½ pounds of fat, 3¼ inches off her waist, 2¼ inches off her hips, and 3½ inches off her thighs in six weeks.

When you do make a dietary change to better yourself remember one thing; you are doing it for you and no one else. I tell clients all the time to be selfish and that they should never let anyone make them feel guilty for doing what they feel is the right thing for them. When you decide to better yourself by improving your dietary habits you are actually doing everyone around you a favor. As Mark Twain once said, "Few things are harder to put up with than the annoyance of a good example." Eventually your example will spread and others will want to follow you… right after they stop kicking and screaming.

What Is A Diet?

As you reach for your second helping of triple chocolate layer cake at the family picnic everything is ok, because you announce that starting tomorrow "I am going to start my new diet." You might as well be saying, "I'm going to food jail." You laugh because you know it's true. The word diet has been hijacked. It is synonymous with voluntarily and temporarily restricting your freedom to eat whatever you want and as much as you want in order to lose weight. This is why "diets" don't work—you fail to understand what a diet really is.

Whenever the restaurant server asks me if I would like dessert, I respond, "No thanks, I'm on a diet." The server looks confused. I don't look like I should be on a diet. Diets are for fat people, right? Wrong! I simply tell the server, "Even though the Death by Chocolate Cake, Mile High Apple Pie, and Googhy Caramel Cheesecake you are waving in my face look delicious, they are not part of my diet." My point is, everyone is on a diet—all the time. Obese people are on a diet. Slender people are on a diet. The origin of the word diet means "way of living." Your diet consists of all the different foods you eat to nourish your body. Some people have a diet that is nourishing and well suited for being lean, energetic, and healthy. Most do not.

It's true; "diets" don't work. A *diet* does. That is, a diet of foods that you are naturally adapted to thrive on—primarily fresh fruits and vegetables. A diet is part of your identity. It is who you are and how you live, constantly. A diet does not have a starting and finishing line. It is not something you go "on" and "off." So why do you oscillate between diets?

Willpower vs. Discipline

Jack Lalanne was asked, "Do you ever splurge?" He responded, "Never. I've got a conscience you wouldn't believe." I disagree. He has *discipline* you wouldn't believe. This comes from years and years of practice.

"Willpower doesn't work," Dr. Lynn Seiser says. "Willpower is often short-lived. It is a burst of motivation and good intention without really learning and practicing any new skills. Discipline is the daily practice of new skills whether you have the willpower to or not; you just do it."

Face the facts. It's easy to go on a diet. It's easy to stay on it for several weeks. The weight loss you experience gives you the motivation to continue, that is, until the going gets tough. Then you cave. Why? You were committed to the goal of looking great, but you did not commit to the discipline it would take to get there and stay there. It was willpower that carried you, but willpower alone will not take you where you want to be. To keep going, to avoid being another yo-yo dieter statistic, and to succeed at being lean requires that you over learn the behaviors that keep you looking and feeling great all the time.

In the spring of 2008 Laura enrolled in my six-week

fat loss program. She lost 14 ½ pounds of fat, 2 ⅝" off her waist, 1 ¾" off her hips, 3 ½" off her thighs, and gained one pound of lean body mass in six weeks. She looked and felt great, and everyone noticed. But it's what happened after the program that made me so happy for Laura.

Many times I hear fat loss program participants remark, "I can do this for six weeks." At that moment I know they have failed before they even start. They are not thinking correctly. They want to be a rock star but don't want to practice playing the guitar. It's frustrating and mind-boggling, but after six weeks many people will look and feel better than they have in a long time, and then immediately go right back to their old lifestyle.

The point of my fat loss program is to teach people the skills necessary to be lean and vibrant forever, not for just six weeks. Remember, discipline is the daily practice of those skills whether you have the willpower to or not. Behavioral psychologists say it takes 100 days of practice to make a behavior automatic, and the more you practice the better. This is what Laura did.

Laura finished the fat loss program on April 22, 2008. She would continue to exercise under my supervision, but she was on her own with the new dietary skills. On June 25 of that same year I emailed her and asked how her results were holding up and she replied "Great! I am sticking to good food and lots of water." She said her body was still changing so I suggested she come in for another round of photos and measurements. She agreed but told me the bathing suit she wore for her initial set of photos was long gone. Her body had changed so much it didn't fit anymore. Nice problem to have.

On July 3, 2008 Laura came in for her photos and measurements. To my surprise, Laura had lost an additional seven pounds of body fat, ⅝" off her waist, 1 ⅛" off her hips and 4 ⅛" off her thighs while gaining another pound and a half of lean body mass. It was now almost 11 weeks since she had completed the program and she was still changing. And keep in mind that during that stretch of time she was only able to come in for three workouts under my supervision. Like I told you before, it's all about the diet.

Laura was now about a size six. I saw her three more times in September, then life got in the way and I have not seen her since, but I keep in touch to see how she is doing. On March 24, 2009, almost one year after completion of the fat loss program, I asked Laura how she was doing and she wrote, "I'm still a size six." She was still practicing the same skills she had learned during the program. She was still exercising her discipline. This way of life was now part of her identity.

Laura is on a diet. This is now her way of living.

What to Eat

Eating is a confusing subject. That is by design. The more confused you are the easier it is to manipulate your choices. That being said, you might think that I would have a lot to say about eating. I don't. In fact, I think the first line of a January 28, 2007 *New York Times* article title "Unhappy Meals" says it best: "Eat food, not too much, mostly plants."

Well, what is food? In response to the question "What is your diet like?" Jack Lalanne answered, "If man makes it, I don't eat it." There you go. Food comes from the earth, not from the mind of a food scientist. Eat as many whole, fresh, unprocessed foods as you want, preferably in their natural state. Don't eat manmade, heavily processed and denatured food-like substances. Eat what nature provides; you can't go wrong, and always remember, nothing tastes as good as feeling great all the time feels. However, it's easier said than done. The deck is stacked against you.

In a 2009 *New York Times* article titled "How the Food Makers Captured Our Brains," author Tara Parker-Pope describes how Dr. David A. Kessler, former head of the Food and Drug Administration and best known for taking on the tobacco industry with his accusation that cigarette makers intentionally manipulated nicotine content to make their products more addictive, wonders why he is helpless against a chocolate chip cookie. Dr. Kessler asks, "Why does that chocolate chip cookie have such power over me? Is it the cookie, the representation of the cookie in my brain? I spent seven years trying to figure out the answer." His research lead to his book, *The End of Overeating: Taking Control of the Insatiable American Appetite.*

Parker-Pope describes Kessler's premise: "When it comes to stimulating our brains, individual ingredients aren't particularly potent. But by combining fats, sugar, and salt in innumerable ways, food makers have essentially tapped into the brain's reward system, creating a feedback loop that stimulates our desire to eat and leaves us wanting more and more even when we're full." He also describes how food scientists "work hard to reach the precise point at which we derive the greatest pleasure from fat, sugar, and salt" in an effort to reach the "bliss point."

It may take a while to get used to, but if you want to be lean, vibrant, and look your best, avoid the things that come in a bag, box, or can. Eat from the earth; this is the best way to optimize your physique and overall health. But just in case you don't believe me, again consider the epigenetics at work here. In his book *Body by Science*, Dr. Doug McGuff illustrates the importance of food choices:

If you undertake the type of behavior that results in a hormonal balance that points to leanness, you will create a nutrient partitioning that favors lean body tissue over fatty tissue. The converse is also true: if you eat a lot of refined foods that are easily digestible and produce elevated insulin levels and excess storage of glycogen and body fat, you will lose your insulin sensitivity on your muscle cells. At the same time, insulin sensitivity on the fat cells is preserved, and you end up having nutrient partitioning that results directly in body fat storage. This leads to a condition known as "internal starvation."

Feed your muscles, not your fat. By eating from the earth you will flip on genetic switches that will stomp down a metabolic path favoring lean tissue over body fat. In other words, eating the right foods begets more eating of the right foods. Eating right will create a cycle that works for you, not against you.

Trust yourself. Add the right diet to the right exercise and you will be thrilled.

CHAPTER THIRTEEN

Beware of Bootcamp

On February 29, 2008 Laura O. (not to be confused with Laura in Chapter 12) began competing in a 12-week company-sponsored physical transformation contest, and she wanted to win. In order to give her an advantage in the competition, Laura hired, as she put it, "a VERY big name trainer who trains famous fitness models." Every two weeks they would have a conference call and he would update her food and workout schedule based on her results. "He gave me a fairly low-carbohydrate, high protein diet and he would take carbohydrates away every two weeks. So my carbohydrate and calories were dropping continually," Laura said.

Four days a week she would do a one-hour weight training circuit. This consisted of doing one set of a group of two or three exercises in rapid succession, then immediately doing five minutes of cardio, then immediately back to another set of the exercises, then five minutes of cardio, and so on until she completed three rounds. After that she would move on to another group of two or three exercises and repeat the same procedure. She would alternate between lower and upper body exercises on different days.

At the beginning of her training program she was taking in 1,400 calories a day. In addition to the weight training circuit mentioned above, Laura did 20 minutes of cardio in the morning and evening four days a week. By week eight Laura was consuming about 1000 calories daily. She was still doing the weight circuit, and was now up to 45 minutes of cardio in the morning and evening six days a week. All of this was accomplished despite a small amount of dietary carbohydrates – ⅛ cup of oatmeal and a salad each day.

"I finally quit at about nine weeks," Laura said. "You cannot imagine how exhausted I was. I was getting no sleep because I had to get up to do cardio in the morning and my evening cardio made it hard to fall asleep. I wasn't getting nearly enough calories. A lot of my coworkers thought I was looking ill, but my closest friend was the one who was really worried about me. She was the one who convinced me to stop and just do a reduced version of the program."

So at week nine Laura went her own way and followed a reasonable diet, did cardio once a day, and continued the weight circuit.

Now, there is something you should know about Laura. She is a 46 year-old mother of two who works a high stress corporate job. She is tough, determined, and a hard worker. She is no sissy. And yet, this boot camp pace reduced her to mush. Was it really necessary? No.

Now let's move to 2009.

A Research Project is Born

In February 2009, Laura came to visit me and asked if I would train her for the 2009 contest. I accepted her request. But this was going to be more than just another series of exercise sessions. A research project was shaping up.

Laura told me that one of the perks of competing in this contest was body composition testing via underwater weighing, which has long been considered the gold standard for body composition measurement. The same company that did the testing in the previous year would also be doing the testing this year. Laura still had her results from the year before, so the scientist in me was excited about the opportunity to compare the results from two polar opposite approaches to body transformation, and have body composition analysis provided by an independent third party.

In 2008, Laura began the contest with a body weight of 152.5 pounds and fat mass of 41.1 pounds. In 2009, Laura began the contest with a body weight of 153 pounds and fat mass of 41.3 pounds. As you can see, her starting point for both years was nearly identical.

The Plan

On February 18, 2009, Laura came in for her photos, measurements, and marching orders. Her plan was the following:

Follow a moderate-calorie high carbohydrate diet. Calories would begin at 1,100 for the first two weeks; increase to 1,300 in week three then descend by 100 through week six. In week seven go back to the beginning and repeat the schedule through to week twelve.

Absolutely **no cardio!** In fact, I told Laura to do no other activity outside of my supervision. Leisurely walking was all right, but only leisurely.

Rest more. Be in bed by 9 p.m. each night. Sleep as late as possible in the morning without getting in trouble at work. Take naps during the day if needed.

High intensity strength training *once a week* under my supervision.

Drink one gallon of water each day. Live your life and be happy.

The Exercise

Laura's exercise was very intense, but very brief. Her first three workouts consisted of five basic exercises that taxed all the major muscle groups in the body. She performed a leg press, pull down, chest press, hip extension, and lateral raise exercise. From the beginning of the first exercise to the end of her last exercise, the elapsed time of her workouts was:

Workout 1 – 8 minutes 25 seconds
Workout 2 – 8 minutes 10 seconds
Workout 3 – 8 minutes 15 seconds

As her calories began to decline in the fourth and fifth

weeks, I reduced Laura's workout to three basic exercises. I did this because I didn't want to add the stress of exercise to the stress her body was going to feel from a calorie reduction. I knew she would have a better chance at losing fat if we kept her body as comfortable as possible. In the sixth week when her calories went to the lowest point, I reduced Laura's workout to two exercises. If this sounds counterintuitive, you have to remember that there is only so much stress your body can cope with. When your goal is fat loss, a little stress is good, but too much can be counterproductive. So the elapsed times of her next three workouts were the following:

Workout 4 – 3 minutes 55 seconds
Workout 5 – 4 minutes 26 seconds
Workout 6 – 2 minutes 45 seconds

That was all the exercise Laura did for the first six weeks, a total of 36 minutes.

At the midpoint of the contest in 2008, the body composition analysis revealed that Laura had lost 10.3 pounds of body fat. The problem was she had also lost three pounds of lean body mass; not a surprise with the type of pace she was keeping. In 2009, Laura had lost 5.7 pounds of body fat, but gained 0.3 pounds of lean body mass. All of her weight loss was fat loss. So I ask you, is it better to lose 10.3 pounds of fat and lose three pounds of lean body mass OR lose 5.7 pounds of body fat and gain 0.3 pounds of lean body mass? You may be inclined to think that Laura's results were better in 2008 because she lost more fat. That is understandable, but as you will soon learn, what happens to your fat mass is only part of the picture. You must account for what happens to your lean body mass.

At this point I received an email from Laura: "It appears right now that I am at about the same (or better?) results this time, but I am not killing myself and I am not feeling bad. I really can't explain to you what a mess I was towards the end of last time. I was mentally foggy and very grumpy. This time I feel fine and could keep going like this forever." And on she went.

The next six weeks were basically a repeat of the first six weeks. Laura was now much stronger and using much heavier weight loads which reduced the time of each individual exercise and consequently the overall length of her workouts. Laura's workout times were 6:20, 6:14, 3:49, 3:32, 1:34, and 1:56. At the end of the 12-week program her total exercise time was approximately 61 minutes, a long way from the endless hours she logged in 2008. She finished the contest feeling great and received many compliments on her appearance. I received a note from Laura that said "I certainly had a lot more fun this time!!!"

Proof is in the Pudding

At the end of the contest we looked at the numbers. In 2008 Laura used the bootcamp approach that required approximately 7-13 hours of exercise each week and lost

14.2 pounds of fat, but lost 2 pounds of lean body mass. That's bad weight loss. In 2009 Laura used my minimalist approach that required a total of 61 minutes of exercise in 12 weeks and lost 14.6 pounds of fat while her lean body mass remained virtually unchanged. Her weight loss was all fat loss in 2009. That's good weight loss.

At this point I posed the question to Laura, "Do you still think you need a lot of exercise?" She replied, "Believe me; I have been thinking *a lot* about the answer to your question." Then she continued by saying, "The exercise was definitely easier. I was so tired last year that I felt bad all the time and didn't have time for a social life. As for the diet, I was hungry all the time last year and this year has been relatively painless and delicious. And, most importantly, I was effectively at the same place this time last year and *everybody* commented that I needed to stop losing weight because I looked so bad. I have not had that this time, the difference being that I have been eating healthy, not low carbohydrate, and doing a reasonable amount of exercise and getting rest. I was literally killing my body last year for the same result."

Later on as I was casually looking over the numbers I realized that Laura's body weight change for both years was nearly identical, yet in 2009 no one thought she looked terrible and needed to stop losing weight.

Why?

Was it the change in her body weight that was responsible for her unhealthy appearance in 2008? She lost 16 pounds of body weight that year. Shouldn't a loss of 16 pounds have made her look better? In 2009 she lost 15.5 pounds of body weight, yet she looked vibrant and felt great.

The point is losing body weight will not necessarily make you look better, especially when you lose lean body mass. So why did Laura's appearance alarm people in 2008? The answer is simply too much stress, too little rest, and a loss of lean body mass. Do you remember the number one biomarker of aging I mentioned in Chapter 2? It is muscle mass. When your muscles wither away your body ages in fast forward. Although Laura did succeed at losing weight in 2008, she did so at the expense of her health and appearance.

The moral of this story is that you do not have to beat yourself up to look and feel great. In fact, just the opposite is necessary for the results you want. Make your body think life is a bed of roses. Send no threatening signals. Sleep more, drink more water, eat healthy food, get the right amount of exercise, and relax. This will unleash the incredible healing power of your body, and it will make you look fantastic.

Losing fat, gaining muscle, and feeling fantastic should not require suffering. When you do it right it should feel like you are cheating. Do the opposite of what you think you should do and you will get better results every time.

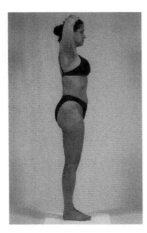 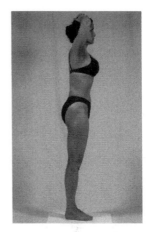

Figure 8 Laura's transformation over 12 weeks with only 61 minutes of exercise. During that time, Laura lost 5 inches off her mid-section, 1 ¼ inches off her hips, and 3 ¼ inches off her thighs.

CHAPTER FOURTEEN

A Gold Brick

"Imagine you are on a hiking trip through some rugged desert terrain. You see a figure in the distance. It's an old man, bearded and half-naked, on hands and knees, with his fingers clawing at the hard, sandy earth. You ask, '*What are you doing?*'

Old Man: '*I'm digging for gold.*'

You: '*How long have you been at it?*'

Old Man: '*Weeks — months maybe. It's painfully slow work.*'

"You notice the old man's bloody fingers, his raw and callused knuckles. You say, '*But listen! Digging with your bare hands is a pretty inefficient way to prospect for gold. That hole's only a couple of feet deep. Let me loan you my shovel.*'

"You reach into your backpack, pull out a lightweight, tempered-edge spade, and drive it into the ground. Then, you show the man how he can break and scoop the hard sand much more efficiently. In less than five minutes you have demonstrated to the old fellow that he can make more progress in a few moments than he could in a month of using his bare hands.

"Then, an amazing thing happens. That old man's eyes fill with hate and his face flushes angrily. He charges at you and grabs the shovel from your hands. He's now preparing to throw the shovel, or perhaps even try to beat you with it.

"You quickly retreat, and get the hell out of the old man's range, as the shovel comes crashing down behind you on the hard sand.

"If you return to that rugged location in the desert a year later, what would you expect to see that old man doing? Would he be using the shovel properly and have holes as big as school buses spread over the immediate and adjacent surroundings? No, absolutely not! Instead, the prospector would be at that same spot—with a somewhat bigger hole—still digging with his even-more-callused fingers. And there, in plain sight, only a few yards away . . . would be the unused, and now rusty, shovel."

This parable was told at many Nautilus® seminars by the brilliant and late inventor of Nautilus® exercise equipment, Arthur Jones. It reflects the reaction he would often receive to teaching people a better way to exercise. Why share this with you? Mark Twain said, "What gets us into trouble is not what we don't know. It's what we know for sure that just ain't so." Most of what you have been taught about losing weight and looking attractive "just ain't so," and it's getting you into trouble. There is a better way. You are holding it in your hands.

This book is about unlearning in order to finally take

your first step toward lasting success. Although I realize that it's natural for you to be unsure and fearful of change, if you are willing to embrace what I have taught you and put my recommendations to the test, I promise you will never go back. Instead of digging for gold all you have to do is put out your hand. I am going to hand you a gold brick. The following recommendations for how to proceed after reading this book will change your life in more ways than you can imagine.

Start a High Intensity Strength Training Program

Make this priority number one. This is the most important thing you can do for yourself right now. It doesn't matter what kind of shape you are in or what your health status is right now. Getting stronger will have your muscle to fat ratio moving in the right direction. This success will then motivate you to practice a wide array of healthy behaviors that will feed the desire for more healthy behavior. I can't stress this point enough; if you choose to make no other change in your life, at least make strength training a regular part of your lifestyle.

I realize the phrase "high intensity strength training" may sound intimidating, but the actual act is not. In fact, it's quite exhilarating. All you need is a little guidance to get you started. Visit my website at WWW.STTLW.COM to learn how you can implement a strength training program in your gym or at home and to watch videos of people performing high intensity strength training.

Don't Be Cheap. Buy Yourself a Body Composition Monitor

Get rid of that old bathroom scale. You won't be watching your weight anymore, at least not the same way you used to. It is now essential that you know what is happening to your body composition. To see what is happening to the fat and muscle content of your body I recommend that you purchase a body composition monitor from the Tanita Corporation (www.TANITA.COM). I have used the BC-553 Ironman Body Composition Monitor for the past four years and it has served me well. The cost is $120. There are plenty of other options available but you need to make sure the scale will at the very least tell you body fat percentage, muscle mass, and body water percentage. For even more information, the BC-558 gives you all the readings you need in segments, for example it will tell you how much fat and muscle you have in your right leg or your left arm. The cost is $300, but I think you are worth it.

The other thing you are going to stop doing is getting on the scale every day. It isn't necessary. I do not recommend that you check yourself more frequently than once a month. Remember, you are interested in results. They take time to appear. Fat loss and muscle gain does not occur on a day-to-day basis, at least not enough to register on a body composition monitor. However you decide to do it, take your measurements under the same conditions for comparison confidence.

Please remember, what you are primarily interested in is how your changes trend over time, not fretting about the accuracy of the numbers. For the fun of it, plug your readings into a spreadsheet graph and put in a trend line or do it by hand on a piece of graph paper. If after one year your measurements show a downward trend in body fat percentage you are doing something right.

After years of using a body composition monitor, I have become aware of a few nuances that can be helpful when interpreting your results. If you have questions about how to track and interpret your results please contact me.

Get More Sleep

This is the most important thing you can do for your overall health and well being.

Harmonize with the light and dark cycles of the earth. When it gets dark at night, turn off the lights and go to bed. When the sun comes up, get out of bed. In *Lights Out*, author T.S Wiley says, "Sleep as many hours as you can without getting fired or divorced." By the way, I highly recommend that you read *Lights Out*. Although I am not in total agreement with all of the dietary recommendations, the authors provide some helpful guidelines and a fantastic explanation of what will happen to you when you don't sleep enough. This book will not only improve your muscle to fat ratio, but it may also save your life.

Hydrate Yourself

Seventy-five percent of the population is chronically dehydrated. That probably includes you. Whenever I talk about hydration clients say, "Oh, I drink a lot of water." Well, there's a lot more to it than that. Yes, drink a lot of water, especially if you eat a lot of processed foods, but the best way to hydrate your system is to eat plenty of high water content foods and eliminate dehydrating lifestyle habits. The most common habits are too much salt, seasonings, alcohol, sodas, and coffee. It doesn't matter how much water you drink when you take in stimulants and toxins that dehydrate your body.

Eat From the Earth

All right, I give in. I know you're dying for some specific dietary recommendations, but before I give those to you I need to say something. I've heard just about every excuse there is for not eating better quality food, so before I go any further let me first say that I don't expect ANYONE to implement the following dietary changes overnight. If you so choose, it will most likely take a long time for you to make these changes. I know; it took me 10 years to do it.

Keep in mind that the following recommendations are for *optimizing* your results in the shortest amount of time. Even if you attempt to make small changes in the direction

I am pointing you, I promise you will begin to lose fat and feel markedly better. It will take you a longer time to get where you want to be, but at least you will be heading in the right direction. It's the direction, not the speed with which you get there that is most important.

At least 50 percent of your diet should consist of fresh, uncooked fruits and vegetables. Although I could go on and on about all the benefits of eating such nutritious food, nothing I write would make one bit of difference in your life. You need to do it and experience the benefits for yourself.

Consider meat as a side dish rather than a main course and aim to consume it less often. When you eat it go for the best quality possible. Beef should be grass-fed only, fish wild-caught and fresh, and chicken that is truly free range and allowed to eat its natural diet of bugs, wild grains, wild grass, and anything else it may be able to catch in a field.

Do your homework.

You would be best served if you avoid all grains—rice, corn, and especially wheat—in any form. Anything with flour in it will create an acidic environment within your body and tear you apart from the inside out. Have you ever wondered why so many people have digestive disorders? Grains play a large role. Although going gluten-free is a good place to start, it's not a complete step in the right direction. Strive to avoid grains altogether. They are very addicting and will keep you fat and unhealthy.

For goodness sake, avoid dairy products like they are the plague. You are an adult human, not a baby cow. Cow's milk does *not* do a human body good.

If you would like a great tip, here is one that works every time. If you like to eat breakfast, eat nothing but fruit until noon. Eat as much as you want. The reason? Your body is in detoxification high gear in the morning hours.

Anything you put in your body that takes a lot of energy to digest, such as high fat and protein type foods, will slow down your body's ability to keep you looking and feeling young. Fruit is digested quickly and cleanly and will not interfere with the housecleaning process. This tip has prompted many clients to tell me "Brian, that was a great piece of advice." Give it a try and let me know how it works out for you.

If you would like to know how you should eat for optimum health and body composition, I strongly recommend that you read *The 80/10/10 Diet* by Dr. Douglas Graham. You can also visit my blog at BRIANMURRAY.WORDPRESS. COM that includes food and exercise advice.

Ditch the Cardio

Cardio is the proverbial turd in the punch bowl. Forget it. I promise you won't miss it. The only thing you will regret is that you didn't do this sooner. Be an active person but don't use cardio to improve your body.

Relax and Live Your Life Without Fear

Every day messages come at you from a million directions designed to scare the pants off you and create even more confusion in your mind. I hope I have given you at least a little more confidence to ignore most of popular weight loss culture. Although I don't expect you to believe a word I say, I sure hope you attempt to understand what I'm teaching you. The best way to do this is by *doing*, and not making excuses. You may think that my advice is good for others who don't have as far to go, for those who only need to tone up, for those who are younger than you or who have better genes than you. Nothing could be further from the truth. If you have a body, the information in this book can work for you.

I used to doubt the same things that I am promoting in this book. Like you, I was fearful of change. However, once I set my mind to explore something different and honestly immersed myself completely in a new way of thinking, I quickly started to see through all the illusions that had been holding me back.

Your anxiety and fear of change is normal, but it can keep you spinning your wheels. What I have taught you will allow you to relax in the cloak of confidence that these new thought patterns provide. Make your muscles stronger, eat right, get plenty of sleep, and relax. Everything will fall right into place.

Endnotes

Chapter 1 – Bad Weight Loss

1. Gina Kolata, "Diet and Lose Weight? Scientists Say 'Prove It!" *New York Times*, January 4, 2005, www.nytimes.com/2005/01/04/health/nutrition/04fat.html (accessed October 24, 2009).
   See *Wikipedia*. Definition of dehydration, http://en.wikipedia.org/wiki/Dehydration (accessed October 24, 2009).

2. Gina Kolata, "Longing to Lose at a Great Cost," *New York Times*, January 4, 2005, www.nytimes.com/2005/01/04/health/04fatb.html (accessed October 24, 2009).

3. David B. Allison, et al. "Weight Loss Increases and Fat Loss Decreases All Cause Mortality Rate: Results From Two Independent Cohort Studies," *International Journal of Obesity and Related Metabolic Disorders* 6 (June 1999):603-11.

4. Timothy S. Church, et al. "Changes in Weight, Waist Circumference and Compensatory Responses with Different does of Exercise Among Sedentary, Overweight

Postmenopausal Women," *PloS ONE* 4(2): e4515.doi:10.1371/journal.pone.0004515.

5. Dr. Lynn Seiser (Identity Therapist) in discussion with author.

Chapter 2 – Bad Weight Loss

1. Ellington Darden, *Body Defining*. (McGraw Hill, 1996).

2. William Evans and Irwin H Rosenberg, *Biomarkers: The 10 Keys to Prolonging Vitality*. (New York: A Fireside Book published by Simon and Shuster, 1991).

Chapter 5 – Walking Is Not Exercise

1. F.M. Ivey, et al, "Effects of Strength Training and Detraining on Muscle Quality: Age and Gender Comparisons," *Journal of Gerontology: Biological Sciences* 55A no.3 (March 2000): B152-157.

2. Edward J. Jakowski, *Hold It! You're Exercising Wrong* (New York: Fireside Publishing, 1995), 75.

Chapter 6 – Life in a Fool's Paradise

1. Average size female data can be viewed at the following CDC website link: http://www.cdc.gov/nchs/fastats/bodymeas.htm (accessed November 3, 2009).

    See the definition of basal metabolic rate at http://health.discovery.com/tools/calculators/basal/basal.html (accessed October 24, 2009).

2. Gina Kolata, "Putting Very Little Weight in Calorie Counting Methods," *New York Times*, December 20, 2007, http://www.nytimes.com/2007/12/20/health/nutrition/20BEST.html (accessed October 24, 2009).

3. John Cloud, "Why Exercise Won't Make You Thin." *Time*, August 9, 2009, http://www.time.com/time/health/article/0,8599,1914857,00.html (accessed October 24, 2009).

Chapter 7 – You Eat Too Much

1. KE Ebersole, et al, "Energy Expenditure and Adiposity in Nigerian and African American Women," *Obesity* 9 (September 2008): 2148-54.

2. LiveScience Staff, "Study: Exercise Won't Cure Obesity," *LiveScience*, January 6, 2009, http://www.livescience.com/health/090106-exercise-obesity.html (accessed October 24, 2009).

3. John Cloud, "Why Exercise Won't Make You Thin," *Time*, Sunday, August 9, 2009, http://www.time.com/time/health/article/0,8599,1914857,00.html (accessed October 24, 2009).

4. Fran Lowry, "The Obesity Epidemic in the US Is Due Solely to Increased Food Intake," *The Heart.Org*, May 14, 2009, http://www.theheart.org/article/970183.do (accessed October 24, 2009).

Chapter 9 – Exercise in Futility

1. David Sheff, "Whatever Happened to Jane Fonda

in Tights," *New York Times*, February 8, 2007, www.nytimes.com/2007/02/08/fashion/08Fitness. html (accessed October 24, 2009).

2. TS Wiley and Bent Formby, *Lights Out: Sleep, Sugar, and Survival* (New York: Pocket Books, a division of Simon and Schuster, 2000), 13-14.

3. Gina Kolata, "*Runner's High? Endorphins? Fiction, Some Scientists Say,*" *New York Times*, May 21, 2002, http://www.nytimes.com/2002/05/21/ health/runner-s-high-endorphins-fiction-some-scientists-say.html (accessed October 24, 2009).

4. TS Wiley, *Lights Out*, 12-13.

Chapter 10 – You Can't Make Your Heart Stronger

1. Arthur C. Guyton, *Textbook of Medical Physiology*, (Philadelphia, PA: W.B. Saunders Company, 1981), 158.
    EL Fox, RW Bowers, ML Foss, *The Physiological Basis of Physical Education and Athletics*. (Dubuque, Iowa: Wm. C. Brown Publishers, Fourth Edition, 1988), 250.

2. BD Charash, *Heart Myths* (New York: Penguin, 1992), 223.

3. G.A Sheehan, M.D. "Take the Muscles and Run," *Physician and Sports Medicine* 9 (May 1981): 35.

4. H. Solomon. *The Exercise Myth* (New York: Bantam Books, 1986), 21-22.
    H Klitgaard et al., "Function, Morphology and

Protein Expression of Aging Skeletal Muscle:
A Cross Sectional Study of Elderly Men
With Different Training Backgrounds," *Acta
Physiol Scand* 1 (September 1990): 41-54

Chapter 11 – Real Health Insurance

1. Wayne Wescott, "Increased Muscle Equals
    Increased Metabolic rate Equals Weight Loss,"
    FitCommerce.com, http://www.fitcommerce.
    com/BLUEPRINT/Increased-Muscle-=-
    Increased-Resting-Metabolic-Rates-=-Weight-
    Loss_page.aspx?pageId=744&tabIndex=5&
    portalId=2 (accessed October 24, 2009).

2. "Lifting weights Keep Overweight at Bay"
    originally appeared on the website *HealthDay
    News* on March 3, 2006. The article can be
    accessed from http://www.medicineonline.
    com/news/10/7838/Lifting-Weights-Keeps-
    Overweight-at-Bay.html as of October, 2009.

Chapter 12 – Religion, Sex, Politics, and…Diet

1. Michael Pollan, *The Omnivores Dilemma:
    A Natural History of Four Meals* (New
    York: The Penguin Press, 2006), 300.

2. Dr. Lynn Seiser (Identity Therapist)
    in discussion with author.

3. Michael Pollan, "Unhappy Meals," *New York
    Times*, January 28, 2007, http://www.nytimes.
    com/2007/01/28/magazine/28nutritionism.t.html

(accessed October 24, 2009).

4. Tara Parker-Pope, "How the Food Makers Captured Out Brains" *New York Times*, June 23, 2009, http://www.nytimes.com/2009/06/23/health/23well.html (accessed October, 24, 2009).

5. "The Fountain of Youth," toyourhealth.com, December 2007, 8-11.

6. Kessler, David A, *The End of Overeating: Taking Control of the Insatiable American Appetite* (New York: Rodale Books, 2009).

7. Doug McGuff and John Little, *Body by Science: A Research Based Program to Get the Results You Want in 12 Minutes a Week* (New York: McGraw Hill, 2008), 199. Also see Chapters 8 and 9 for a discussion of epigenetics.

Chapter 14 – A Gold Brick

1. Ellington Darden, *The Nautilus Body Building Book* (Chicago: Contemporary Books, 1982), 2. TS Wiley and Bent Formby, *Lights Out: Sleep, Sugar, and Survival* (New York: Pocket Books, a division of Simon and Schuster, 2000), 164.

Bibliography

Allison, David B., et al. "Weight Loss Increases and Fat Loss Decreases All Cause Mortality Rate: Results From Two Independent Cohort Studies." *The International Journal of Obesity and Related Metabolic Disorders* 23, no. 6 (June 1999): 603-11.

Charash, BD. *Heart Myths.* New York: Penguin, 1992.

Church TS, Martin CK, Thompson AM, Earnest CP, Mikus CR, et al. "Changes in Weight, Waist Circumference and Compensatory Responses with Different Doses of Exercise among Sedentary, Overweight Postmenopausal Women." *PLoS ONE* 4(2): e4515. doi:10.1371/journal.pone.0004515.

Cloud, John. "Why Exercise Won't Make You Thin." *Time,* August 9, 2009. http://www.time.com/time/health/article/0,8599,1914857,00.html (accessed October 24, 2009).

Darden, Ellington. *Body Defining.* McGraw Hill, 1996.

———*The Nautilus Bodybuilding Book.* Lincolnwood (Chicago), Illinois: Contemporary Books, 1982.

Discovery Health, definition of basal metabolic rate. *http://health.discovery.com/tools/calculators/basal/basal. html* (accessed October 24, 2009).

Ebersole, KE., et al. "Energy Expenditure and Adiposity in Nigerian and African American Women." *Obesity* 9 (September 2008): 2148-54.

Evans, William and Rosenberg, Irwin H. *Biomarkers: The 10 Keys to Prolonging Vitality.* New York: Fireside Publishing, 1992.

Fox, EL., Bowers, RW., Foss, ML. *The Physiological Basis of Physical Education and Athletics.* Dubuque, Iowa: Wm. C. Brown Publishers, Fourth Edition, 1988.

Graham, Douglas. The 80/10/10 Diet. Key Largo, Florida: *FoodnSport Press*, 2006.

Guyton, Arthur, C and Hall, John E. *Textbook of Medical Physiology.* Philadelphia, PA: W.B. Saunders Company, 1981.

HealthDay News, original publication of "Lifting Weights Keep Overweight at Bay." March 3, 2006. http://www. medicineonline.com/news/10/7838/Lifting-Weights-Keeps-Overweight-at-Bay.html (accessed October 25, 2009).

Ivey, FM., et al. "Effects of Strength Training and Detraining on Muscle Quality: Age and Gender Comparisons." *Journal of Gerontology: Biological Sciences* 55A no.3 (March 2000): B152-157.

Jakowski, Edward J. *Hold It! You're Exercising Wrong.* New

York: Fireside, 1995.

Kessler, David A. *The End of Overeating: Taking Control of the Insatiable American Appetite.* New York: Rodale Books, 2009.

Klitgaard H., et al. "Function, Morphology and Protein Expression of Aging Skeletal Muscle: A Cross Sectional Study of Elderly Men With Different Training Backgrounds." *Acta Physiologica Scandinavica* 140, no. 1 (September 1990):41-54.

Kolata, Gina. "Diet and Lose Weight? Scientists Say 'Prove It!'" *New York Times,* January 4, 2005. www.nytimes. com/2005/01/04/health/nutrition/04fat.html (accessed October 24, 2009).

——— "*Longing* to Lose at a Great Cost." The *New York Times,* January 4, 2005. www.nytimes.com/2005/01/04/health/04fatb.html (accessed October 4, 2009).

——— "*Putting* Very Little Weight in Calorie Counting Methods." *New York Times,* December 20, 2007. http://www.nytimes.com/2007/12/20/health/nutrition/20BEST.html (accessed October 24, 2009).

——— "*Runner's* High? Endorphins? Fiction, Some Scientists Say." *New York Times,* May 21, 2002. http://www.nytimes.com/2002/05/21/health/runner-s-high-endorphins-fiction-some-scientists-say.html (accessed October 24, 2009).

Little, John and McGuff, Doug. *Body by Science: A Research Based Program to Get the Results You Want in 12 Min-*

utes a Week. New York: McGraw Hill, 2008.

LiveScience Staff. "Study: Exercise Won't Cure Obesity." *LiveScience*, January 6, 2009. http://www.livescience.com/health/090106-exercise-obesity.html.

Lowry, Fran. "The Obesity Epidemic in the US Is Due Solely to Increased Food Intake." *The Heart.Org*, May 14, 2009. http://www.theheart.org/article/970183.do (accessed October 24, 2009).

Parker-Pope, Tara. "How the Food Makers Captured Out Brains." *New York Times*, June 23, 2009. http://www.nytimes.com/2009/06/23/health/23well.html (accessed October, 24, 2009).

Pollan, Michael. *The Omnivores Dilemma: A Natural History of Four Meals*. New York: The Penguin Press, 2006.

———*"Unhappy* Meals." *New York Times*, January 28, 2007. http://www.nytimes.com/2007/01/28/magazine/28nutritionism.t.html (accessed October 24, 2009).

Sheehan, GA., M.D. "Take the Muscles and Run." *Physician and Sports Medicine* 9 (May 1981): 35.

Sheff, David. "Whatever Happened to Jane Fonda in Tights?" *New York Times*, February 8, 2007. www.nytimes.com/2007/02/08/fashion/08Fitness.html (accessed October 24, 2009).

Solomon, H. *The Exercise Myth*. New York: Bantam Books, 1986.

Toyourhealth.com. "The Fountain of Youth." December

2007: 8-11.

Wescott, Wayne. "Increased Muscle Equals Increased Metabolic rate Equals Weight Loss." *FitCommerce. com.* http://www.fitcommerce.com/BLUEPRINT/ Increased-Muscle-=-Increased-Resting-Metabolic-Rates-=-Weight-Loss_page.aspx?pageId=744&tabInd ex=5&portalId=2 (accessed October 24, 2009).

Wikipedia. Definition of cortisol. http://en.wikipedia.org/ wiki/Cortisol (accessed October 24, 2009).

Wikipedia. Definition of dehydration. http://en.wikipedia. org/wiki/Dehydration (accessed October 24, 2009).

Wiley, TS and Formby, Bent. *Lights Out: Sleep, Sugar, and Survival.* New York: Pocket Books, a division of Simon and Schuster, 2000.

Made in the USA
Columbia, SC
29 May 2021